Bedtime Stories for Adults

Ensure you a relaxing and restoring deep sleep to leave anxiety, stress and insomnia out from your

bedroom once for all

reading the best bedtime novels ever

Table of Contents

Sophia's Fear

You feel the tapping of your clean, white shoes on the soles of your feet hitting the ground. You feel the shock of the sole and all the impact on your sole.

A few seconds ago she stepped out of the silver indoor elevator where she felt locked in a refrigerator where she locked up all her patients.

She walks down the long hospital corridor, doesn't understand why that area has to stay in the basement and why she has to work alone every night, although she has vast experience, lately, she has found it hard to be alone there.

She finally arrives at the cream-colored double door where she will be until four in the morning. Pathology, Sophia is a pathologist, every night she has to check the corpses that were admitted that day, following the routine procedure that all dead people have.

During the day they are also treated, but this city does not rest and from Harlem, there are always corpses arriving, many of them murdered in terrible ways.

When she enters the room where she will have to attend to her patients, she stands at the door, symmetrically arranged there are 8 stretchers, four on each side, with white sheets over bundles of different sizes, men, women, fat and thin, even where there seems to be no body, the body of an old woman rests on the bones, it seems to have died naturally, although she has to do the autopsy anyway.

Sophia has four months with the night shift, she took it because after working the whole day she stayed in bed, looking at the ceiling, not being able to sleep, then, in order not to sleep, she does it at night and deliberately chose the shift that ends at 4 because just at that time she feels the body heavy and where she goes to bed she sleeps until seven, she only needs three hours to recover. This way he has the day completely free.

—"Good night, handsome", Sophia says to a corpse that she uncovered, the first one of the night, is a dark and tall, muscular man, who seems to sleep, and when she details him she discovers three holes in his chest and one just behind his ear.

—How did they kill you? —she asks.

She starts with the skull, takes her tool, and begins to draw a line through the whole area of the head, when she completes the turn, she gently separates the cap and takes out the brain, studies the trajectory of the bullet, takes it out and deposits it in a metal plate.

As she does this, a lighted tape recorder records everything she says out loud.

Then she makes an incision in the whole chest up to the groin, Sophia cannot avoid seeing the crotch of the corpse and smiles and sees the man's face.

—Tremendous waste you were, a pity to meet us in these circumstances.

She checks each organ, takes out the viscera, and extracts the bullets that go to the same place as the first one. One bullet went through the heart, another

10

through the stomach and the last one through the lung. The headshot was not necessary, the first three had been fatal.

When she finishes, she closes the body and leaves it totally clean. Sophia has always been accustomed to treating bodies with respect; the seams she makes are not those horrible ones that all pathologists make, but she makes them with love, as if they were going to heal. When she finishes with the colored man, she covers him with the sheet up to his neck and leaves his face uncovered, as if he were sleeping; it is something she does every night to have the company, during the night she talks to everybody when she sees their names she calls them for him, sometimes she tells them her life, and admits that the dead are the best listeners.

She goes and discovers another body, this one is that of an extremely obese woman who after the autopsy discovers that her immense and greasy heart did not bear her 160 kilos of existence so much and exploded.

The thin old woman, after undergoing the same procedure as the previous ones, discovers that she died from lungs rotten with tobacco smoke, a life of smoking Camel took its toll and now she is a corpse. Therein lies the reason for her thinness.

That is how she discovers bodies, all dead for different reasons, several for murder, some with bullets, others with knives, and one was even in parts because apparently he was attacked with an axe, because she almost had to put together a puzzle to determine.

She sometimes doesn't understand the medical rules that require a body to be autopsied in these circumstances. Why did he die? He was hacked to pieces and there is nothing more to investigate. He was chopped to death, so she makes her report, outlining everything that was chopped in half and what axe it was that probably killed him.

She checks other bodies, one man's neck was slit, and he looks almost blue, because he bled to death. While doing the autopsy, she discovered that he had an immense tumor in his stomach, probably cancer because of the color. If that cut didn't kill him, he would die for natural reasons in not much time. This was noted and recorded.

When she uncovered the penultimate body she stood there, watching the person, detailing each of his features and shaking, worried, afraid, as if going back a long time, to the times when she had chains on her ankles, when she had to ask permission to urinate and give thanks for the plate of food.

On the stretcher, a woman who confirms on the sheet, is only 21 years old, about to turn 22, her face is beautiful, white, with pink lips, expressive eyes, although now she is not very beautiful, because she had bruises all over her face, her left eye is immense, her eyelid looks like a ping pong ball, her mouth is split. With trembling lips, she lifts her lip and sees that she has several broken teeth and a prosthesis. The nose is sideways, a beautiful nose with a Greek profile, small and thin, now it is a piece of pink flesh sideways.

She discovers it little by little, and she sees her firm, thin body, of a young girl of her age, her breasts are bruised, bitten, by her abdomen there are also bruises

12

that look almost black, her legs are cut, her hands are beaten, there are traces of blood under her nails, she takes samples so that they can deduce the DNA of the alleged bloody murderer.

Sophia has not noticed, but she is crying, all the work she starts to do is with great care, with love, checking every part of her, taking notes with her trembling voice. She caresses the young woman's hair, while her lip trembles and she feels very sorry for what happened to her.

—It's over, baby. You are resting from that wretch. I'm so sorry angel, I hope you're in heaven, resting, happy. If there is another life I hope it is better than the one my queen gave you.

She opened her skull with regret to check that her brain was in perfect condition. She began to open her chest and checked it, discovering that inside she had several internal hemorrhages that caused her to die. She takes the report and does everything with the utmost detail so that nothing in her work will prevent the investigation into this poor woman's death from being tarnished.

When she finishes she sits on the floor, crying, and her mind travels back seven years, at the moment she detailed herself, dirty, with tanned skin, with a stench of urine and feces, with the skin of her ankle scalded by a chain and being a victim of her first boyfriend, who took her home with the promise of having a good time alone and was beaten, reduced by the force of the man and in a basement for several months, until finally she was rescued. The boyfriend confronted the police forces and was murdered in front of her.

She was already halfway through college and decided to switch to pathology, where she started and is now. And then a body of a woman in these conditions appeared, it is as if she went back in time to that time when she was kidnapped and raped countless times.

—"It's a very beautiful woman," says the black man, sitting on his stretcher, with the sheet on his legs.

—"I know," says Sophia.

—"I would have shot her in the middle of her eyes. No, it is very easy, I would have beaten him to death with these hands," he shows her his hands, "I would have hit very well."

—"Don't be violent, son," says the old woman who is lying down and only moves her head to speak to Sophia.

—"Thank you for your words," says Sophia.

—My husband once raised his hand to me and I didn't say anything, but I went to the kitchen, I took an iron frying pan in which I fried his eggs with bacon every morning, I went to the couch where he was watching a Lakers game and I hit him on the forehead with it, it was so strong that he was unconscious for two hours, I was scared, I thought I had killed him, but no, he lived 37 more years.

Sophia tells them what she went through.

—It's in the past, baby. Now you are carrying the rhythm of your life. —Says the man.

—"Sometimes we have to go through a little violence," says the obese woman, sitting naked, looking at the woman.

Sophia closes her eyes and remembers her anxiety exercises. When she calmed down she looked at the bodies, they were resting, as always, it was not the first time she had conversations with them and knew a little about life.

When she stood up, the beaten woman looked at her with the only eye she could open, nothing was said. Sophia finished her work with her missing body and returned to where the young woman, this one waiting patiently, had all the time in the world. It was past four in the morning. Sophia felt sleepy, ran to the young woman, and lay down next to her, hugging her. She closed her eyes and fell asleep.

Emma's Mercy

She must have been a social worker for about fifteen years. In all that time she has had to see all kinds of things, people in street conditions, women abused by their husbands and even by their female partners or by their parents or some family member who has custody.

She has had to face violent people who, when they see her, throw her out on the street, because they know that their toxic worlds are coming to bother them. She has even lost her fear of the weapons that some of these men put in her face and threaten her to get out, and she has developed a leathery skin that makes her resist everything.

The only thing she cannot tolerate is seeing depressed children, of those she finds many, most of them in homes of violent parents, some she has to convince them to come out, because their mother has locked them in the closet and they have a latch inside so that she can stay there when dad... screams a lot.

The first case she had to face of this type was that of a boy who had already been hiding in his sister's closet for two hours. His father, in a fit of anger, had beaten the mother to death and then had gone to the closet to try to get the boy out, but he didn't succeed even though he kicked the door several times, the marks were there. The man, if he wanted to, would have passed, perhaps, in the end, in a fit of humanity, decided to spare his son's life and had run away and aimlessly.

Emma had to sit by the door for a long time and talk to the seven-year-old boy to get him to come out, gaining his trust. She did so with a natural talent that in the end the poor boy came out and hugged her and held on to her for about ten minutes. Finally, they took him to an orphanage, where he would have to grow up from now on.

Although Emma behaved like a hero and had handled everything very tactfully, when she finished, when the boy was transferred in a police car, when he turned the corner, she felt a hot liquid rise from her stomach and threw up the oatmeal she had eaten for breakfast.

All night she cried for that boy and for the luck that would touch him, his world was over, his mother dead, his father in prison, alone, if he was lucky he would come out well, if he resented life he could end up being a criminal and a cycle that repeated itself as it happens in the circles he frequented.

Emma also attended to cases of young pregnant women, helped them, gave them advice, and told them that everything would be fine, many of them didn't even have insurance and in the United States, the cradle of the world, medicine was sometimes not so good and if you don't have insurance, you're screwed. Emma was in charge of helping these women in difficult conditions so they could live a little better.

When she arrives at these places where there are people full of vulnerabilities, usually she is in poor neighborhoods, locations that are not visited by tourists visiting the state, she always feels the nauseating smell hitting her nose, poking the bitter stench through her pits and hitting her brain.

Even though she has been doing this for so many years, she does not stop feeling committed and this mistake has cost her her peace of mind. Every night she wakes up restlessly, thinking about the person on duty she is trying to help, thinking about cases from the past, wondering how she has done, if she will be all right, if she fell into drugs again or the children that one thing or another happened to them. Sometimes she can't take it anymore and gets up, goes away, checks in the next day, and many times she appears as an angel to those people who just needed the help of a social worker.

Although everyone loves Emma, no one knows that the poor woman has sacrificed her life to be able to give a little more peace of mind to those people, that day and night she suffers and the salary she receives is nothing compared to all she gives.

She does not rest, until Sundays, after going to mass she goes to some area between her eyebrows and visits that home where she senses or was informed that there are problems, she knows that on Sundays people are at home, that that day she will be able to approach them and tell them the steps to follow or the consequences to face. Her classmates call her "The Crazy One" because she never rests and because every situation she faces has a tenacity that none of her classmates have.

The others do it for the sake of it, as if they were operating a machine, although some have sensitivity, they don't reach Emma's level, the children when they are put in an orphanage, already, they forget about them, when the woman is released from the hands of a man or helped, they turn the page, and they do everything without having any real affection, people who work for pay.

In one of these visits, she arrives at the house that is left in a suburb, the garden looks abandoned, full of plants that have not been pruned for a long time, outside there are a lot of garbage bags and codeine containers. The house seems to be abandoned, it is known that it is not because of the ranchera parked outside, rusty and with the same appearance of the house and the screams that are heard from outside.

Inside is the woman screaming at her husband where he left his coke, to give it to him or he will kill him right now. Emma is right at the door, thinking about whether to knock or not, but at that moment the man opens with violence, he is on his way out, he doesn't want to listen to his wife.

He's a dirty man, he has sores on his face, he smells, and he gets scared when he sees Emma just as she gets scared.

—You see! —The man shouts at his wife, "Because of you, a woman from social work came again. —The man opens the door wide and asks Emma to come in. He goes to the furniture, removes dirty papers and dishes, and clears the once dark green seat for her, but now it is black. Emma sits down hiding her disgust, the house is a den, the walls are not defined by color, and the windows are covered with wooden strips, as if they were protected from a horde of zombies from the outside.

The woman is in the middle of the room, she is very thin, and she wears jeans that fit her big and a cream-colored t-shirt that goes down over one shoulder.

—What does this bitch want? —She asks her husband.

—The usual, to scold us and say that we are bad parents.

The couple starts yelling at each other, pointing at each other and going out into the street, Emma hears beatings, and they fall into violence. She opens her wallet carefully, takes out her cell phone and goes to her company's application, one that has many options and one of them is an emergency button, which she touches when there is danger or she feels that things could get difficult. This alarm warns the police that by tracking it she will arrive at the site soon.

—I'm not going to let you take my son, you bitch, — says the woman who enters screaming and waving her arms.

Emma is surprised, they have a child? She came with the intention of raising awareness and seeking help, but some sometimes don't need help, they must continue to descend into their hells.

A child comes out of one of the rooms, sees Emma hidden, and holds a Mickey Mouse cuddly toy in his arms, extremely dirty just like the child.

The woman shouts at him to go into the room again and the man who is in the garden shouts something to the woman, she cannot stand it anymore and goes out to the street, more blows are heard.

The boy looks at Emma and she signals with a smile, encouraging him to come to her side. The little one comes closer, he is beautiful, he still keeps part of his innocence in those little shiny eyes, Emma grooms him and feels his fingers sticky, the little one smells bad too, surely it has been a long time since he was bathed.

He looks so much like him.

It's called Emma. Whoever talks to him and tells him that soon help will come that he doesn't have to fear.

—"I'm hungry," says the little one in a whisper, "I'm hungry, but I don't tell Mommy because she gets angry, she doesn't like me to be hungry.

Emma swallows thickly and strokes the little one's head. She promises him that everything will be fine.

A siren sounds and a policeman orders them to put their hands where they can see them. Emma hugs the little one and tells him to forgive him, giving him kisses on his filthy head. A patrol car takes the parents away and another car driven by a female policeman takes the little boy to be examined and to define his future.

Emma stands in front of the house, watching the little boy go off to his new life, feeling very sorry for him and remembering, so many memories from nearly twenty years ago. Emma touches her forearms, caresses them, and feels them softly and her skin without any trace of a needle, not even one, anymore.

21

The Candy Store

Every day the ritual is the same, at 5 and 20 Isabella gets up, walks to the bathroom, sits on the toilet and urinates for 25 seconds, cleans herself, gets up and takes the brush she left ready the night before, brushes herself, while looking sleepy in the mirror at her round face, puts on the big bag that covers her up to her knees and goes out to meet the milkman who passes by every day at exactly 5 and 30.

The candy store is exactly in her house, it is attended by a door that opens in the front, but she has access inside the house too, in fact, it is the garage of the house that enabled it as a store and sale of sweets, then apart from these, she sells milk, juices, and other drinks.

The man says good morning to her, runs in with the basket, and prepares everything on-site, leaving her the refrigerator with fresh milk for that day.

Isabella goes back to bed and sleeps for twenty minutes more, when it's almost six o'clock, she gets up, puts on some decent clothes and goes downstairs to open the door, the gate opens and soon after the first customers start arriving, those who take their children to school, those who go to prepare breakfast, at mid-morning the sales calm down and she takes advantage of it to have breakfast and watch some trash show on TV.

At midday she attends to those clients who arrive at the last minute to buy the drink or dessert they will eat after lunch and during the whole afternoon the store is kept alone, except for some child who comes to buy candy or a person who wants to eat something.

At night the movement starts again, people appear to buy everything they enjoy, and children to spend pennies they are given at home. The day goes like this, one after the other. Isabella stays in the same place every day of the year, sits on a chair at the entrance or behind a display case and after lunch she nods her head in dreams.

She runs the whole store and home alone. She has been doing so since her mother died a few years ago. Isabella did not study beyond high school and now she has to work in this business to be able to pay the mortgage and cover her expenses.

Since she runs the store, everyone knows her in the neighborhood, everyone knew her mother and the entire community was at her mother's funeral, dressed in black, while a priest read a word that no one heard and a black sarcophagus waited to be lowered into the ground.

The woman died of old age, sick, diabetic, obese, life took her to the other world and now, Isabella felt alone the weight of having devoted her life to a mother and to a store and a house, she was left alone, without a partner, without children, and with an age that was beginning to weigh on her back and in her soul.

She had missed out on the best years, those of the parties, those of friends, those of having casual sex, that if she had her friends, those of having boyfriends or a formal partner, that would have broken her heart, no one, except those who didn't even look at her.

She only had the store and the friends from the community who every night chatted with her and told her the latest news from the community

Isabella was not ugly. She could not be considered a beauty advertisement, but she did not fit into the ugly bag either, she was slightly obese, but not to the point of making her body ugly, her face was round and friendly, her skin was white, her eyes were blue like those of the waters in the movie The Blue Lagoon, her hair was a light brown and her smile was cared for, for years she had braces.

She wasn't ugly, she was pretty, a normal pretty, one of those that you choose for life.

The problem was that nobody chose her. Nobody was looking for something in her, not even to pass the time. Isabella was that kind of pretty woman that everyone saw as very nice, but up to there.

That hurt her a lot, because she felt she deserved to be loved, and now, without her mother, this loneliness weighed on her more than ever. Although it was not every night that she would fall into sadness, she would often repeat that her bed was too big and she would wake up looking at the cold pillow next to her, imagining that as a child she had often dreamt of seeing a man there next to her, with a beard, sleeping peacefully or waking up when he surrounded her with his arm.

This did not happen. Never.

Isabella was a good-hearted woman, sometimes children would appear with a dollar bill, some coins, or any other money on top and she was a little short of completing what that candy cost and she would give it to him. One day, a girl appeared in the store who she had never seen before, she must have been about seven or eight years old, beautiful, smiling, and with a mischievous look.

—"Lady," said the girl, —is that candy good? —she asked, pointing to a cupcake combined with a brownie.

—Yes, they take it a lot, it's very good. Do you want to buy one?

The girl shook her head.

—And this one? —Now she pointed to another candy with strawberries on top.

The little girl asked prices, information, and all the details, but she didn't finish buying, although she always returned to the delicious brownie that had been calling her since she had entered.

—Don't you have any money? —Isabella asked.

The little girl shook her head and then said

—But you sell such delicious things, or so it seems.

Isabella smiled, stood up, and walked to the window.

—Which one do you want?

—Really?

Isabella nodded.

The little girl pointed to the brownie and Isabella gave it to him, thanked him, and left happily eating it. She knew that the little girl had manipulated her, but she didn't care, she liked the little girl and she thought she was sweet.

The next day the girl appeared, this time she came with a serious face and was holding the hand of a man with a bald spot starting, he had metal-rimmed glasses and a friendly face, the little hair he had left was golden and he had a small belly.

—Hello, can I help you? —Isabella asked.

—Yes, you can. Did my daughter come to buy you candy yesterday?

—Yes, yesterday, why?

—How did you pay her?

There was a brief pause.

—No... she didn't pay me.

—Then why did you give her the candy? —Did she promise to pay you later?

—No, she seemed like a lovely girl, she looked at the candy with such desire that it made me happy to give her one. Is there a problem?

The man's face relaxed and now he looked nicer, she noticed.

—"You are very kind," the man said, —but I am very ashamed that you have to lose your money giving away your merchandise. I will pay you back, my daughter cannot be receiving candy from strangers, let alone abusing the kindness of others.

—I offered to give it to her and no, she doesn't have to pay me anything, I repeat, I gave it to her. You have a lovely little girl.

The little girl who had been quiet all the time and with her eyes fixed on the floor gave the woman a look. She squeezed her father's hand and Isabella thinks she heard him say "ask her name" because immediately afterward the man appeared

—Hello, I'm Bill.

—Isabella, nice to meet you. They're new because I haven't seen them before.

—Yes, we just moved in a few weeks ago. The neighborhood is beautiful.

So, a conversation began to be woven that went on for a while and the little one also joined in and then there were casual visits of "passing by" and then longer, interesting conversations that went on more and more, even accompaniment to closing the business, an invitation to dinner, words that slipped in, flirtations, furtive caresses in the hand and a crush that gradually came. Bill already knew that she had never had a boyfriend and everything was absolutely new to her.

So he seduced her with all his weapons, gave her what she had always dreamed of, an old-fashioned crush that lasted for several dates, until one day, Isabella, tired of waiting, took her man's face and gave him a kiss. The contact of the lips, wet, warm, with the heat of the breaths of each one hitting the skin of the other, achieved the first longed-for kiss. Both gave themselves to a long-awaited kiss that formalized without many words the relationship.

Now the little girl visited the store frequently, he always showed up and they became the family they did not have. Bill was separated, his wife had left him long ago, the little girl adored her father and the two of them were a team. Bill was a journalist, he worked writing columns for various media and always spent time at home. So he soon began to skip days to work at Isabella's house and soon the three of them were under the same roof. That first night, Isabella woke up in the early morning and smiled when she saw her man Bill next to her, wrapped up and naked under the blanket, sleeping peacefully. Bill felt that she was awake and hugged her and they fell asleep, starting a life together. The woman who deserved Bill had appeared and for Isabella, the wait had been worthwhile, next to her was sleeping the love of her life.

The Impossible Design

Since she was a child, she started drawing with her school crayons. While her classmates made abstract drawings like all children do, she drew more mature strokes, not perfect, but superior to any girl her age.

She was good at drawing, when she entered first grade she would draw what she saw, if she had a container, she did it with a lot of symmetry, she drew silhouettes, she did pointillism and she was always fascinated by the commercials where they talked about painting or art and she would stay watching hypnotized the television on the days that they transmitted the art program where they had a painting section.

Her parents noticed this natural talent and enrolled her in drawing courses where she stood out, soon she was so good that she drew better than the teachers and the courses bored her a lot, her parents had to aspire higher and choose expensive and good courses, anyway, for her it was a piece of cake and she learned very easily.

During her adolescence, like every person who has art in her veins, she went through depressive stages, for dressing in black and challenging her parents, she smoked joints, went out with boys, went out with girls, although she did it for pleasure and even as an adult she does it every now and then, she believes in free love and life is not too complicated.

In design and art she gave everything, she was always obsessed with surpassing techniques and others, that's why she worked hard to be better than her teachers, than her bosses, than everyone, and thanks to that she got a job in a huge company where she designs all their brand and carries their image, she earns a great salary, but even though she has this, which could keep her happy, she is not. She feels she can do more than she needs to achieve that design that nobody can. That's why when artificial intelligence was not yet a reality as it is today, she managed to make some designs where she created from scratch faces of people that do not exist, with a luxury of details that looked like hyperrealistic photographs. This served for an artificial intelligence company to call her and help them create a marketing design based on non-existent faces. Today there is advertising where people hold a product and even everything in the image sells the product, but in reality, that person does not exist, he or she comes out of a computer and Olivia was part of this creation, she helped create design patterns of many faces, hair, eyes, wrinkles and folds. Thanks to her contributions there are so many faces in advertising today that do not exist.

This is how other projects came about where Olivia was the designer. Besides guiding many people in the design process, she also trains those who want to learn many of the tricks and is an excellent teacher.

But even though she lives for design, she breathes design, she is an artist who can create something beautiful in moments, she still feels empty, because she has not been able to find that which really satisfies her and that is to be able to make perfect art. The one that immortalizes her, the one that makes her mark history and makes her the prologue of the new era in design.

That is why she has studied design in-depth, more than she knows, she has gone into marketing, thanks to what she has learned with those of artificial intelligence and she has been analyzing how to give life to those false people of advertising.

But one night when she couldn't sleep, feeling the fabric of the blanket stinging her skin, because it bothered her, she ran the fabric, stayed in her nightgown, and looked at the ceiling, and her mind came to what she had been waiting for.

It is as if she had waited for it all her life but could not see it clearly, but now she could. If she achieved that goal she would attain immortality, no one would forget her name, and if she was lucky she would be summoned to name it.

She wanted to invent a new color, the color Olivia. When someone quoted this shade I wanted them to say "that's the color Olivia".

Although I was clear that I was facing a great challenge, because no one could imagine a new color, the basics were known, the secondary ones and the immense range that came out of them, but to bring out a new color I could not, the brain was not capable of that.

So she put that challenge between her eyes, she began to play with colors, she began in the digital world, where she had been working for years, trying out nuances, moving from one mode to another and applying different palettes but she only achieved color pastes that ended up in greys or shades close to black or brown. Because what Olivia wanted was to create a color that was unique, not one more or a dark one like a

31

brown, a black or a dark purple, no, she wanted one as vivid as yellow, like bright green, or orange, she wanted a tone that would dazzle, and for this, she had to employ many techniques in order to achieve it.

But she didn't get it, obviously, that color doesn't exist, or at least the human eye is not capable of perceiving it, or we human beings believe that it doesn't exist because we are not capable of conceiving it.

Olivia was willing to do anything to begin to discover it, every day she became more obsessed, like the man in the book, The Perfume who consumed his life looking for the perfect aroma and that's why he murdered so many women. She began to think that this tone had to be taken from nature because they were natural colors, so she had to look for it in nature itself, so she went to look for it, to investigate it in the plants, trying the nectar of the most colorful flowers, to combine tones, but she only ended up with the sensation of sticky fingers from crushed plants and murky water without a defined color.

For the first time in her life, Olivia found herself before a challenge that she could not solve, always, since she was a little girl she would overcome the challenges with a medium effort, she would surpass her teachers, the people who taught her design, producers, everyone, she always stood out as the best, even her best teachers would end up asking how she was able to achieve a certain task.

Now, looking for the best color of all, the one that nobody has known, not even her, because when a person undertakes some objective, she has in mind what she wants, she visualizes it, she was not able to find that color either, I go around sticks of blind, to see if she is right.

Her search was becoming more and more bizarre, an old shaman tells her that what she knows is what she is looking for, that she has a place to look for it, inside the pyramids of Mexico, in the temple of Kukulkan, Yucatan, she must find a way to enter and get to the bottom, just where they allow visits, then she has to sneak in and look to get to the interior, the real interior, because they say you can't find it, but yes, and just at the bottom, under some huge rocks is what she is looking for.

Olivia, for several days, thinks about the words of the shaman, decides to ask for a vacation she had never taken and with her savings, she leaves for Mexico. She makes several visits with the guides and analyzes every detail on the walks, seeing vulnerabilities in order to get in.

For several nights, she tried to get in, managed to get around the security, and managed to get to the pyramid and study it, but couldn't find a way in.

Finally, when she was about to give up, she discovered that one of the rocks was not fixed with the others, but that one was a huge block, and it was very difficult to get it out. She was not going to give up, with her hands scalded and sore, she finally managed to enter and reach the inside of the pyramid, and her nose was itchy because of the strange smell.

She began to study every detail of the interior, shining a flashlight and seeing things that she had never seen in her life, in any museum or book, objects that she did not know what they were for, extremely strange.

She continued to investigate, descending stairs that seemed eternal, the pyramids were high on the outside, but inside they were extremely deep, every so often she stopped and sharpened her ears, to see if she heard anything, but no, not even insects were inside.

After a while she reached the last chamber of the pyramid, she knew that it was because at the bottom a sarcophagus was waiting, and next to these sealed vessels. She began to open them, inside there was honey that seemed to have just been taken out of the honeycomb and in a giant container, which she found very difficult to open, she found something that as soon as she removed the lid she saw it shining, she no longer needed the flashlight, her mind was opening up to something that no other human being had seen, only she, and that would be the end of it because Olivia never left the pyramid and no one knew that she entered, she simply disappeared.

Cutting Dreams

She has it all, the comfort that a person can seek, a home, a refrigerator with food, school for the children insured, a job in what she likes, a husband with a permanent job for life that will ensure a quiet retirement, health insurance, and a vacation once a year. She lacks nothing.

So why isn't she happy?

Ava can't explain this to herself. She has a hard time sleeping, her husband barely lies down, babbles something, closes his eyes, his breathing calms down, he becomes more serene and within two minutes he's snoring. She has to walk around for a while instead. She has a good time from this and the lack of sleep has become longer and longer. When she sleeps she has an extremely fragile sleep, any movement, sound, even the sound of a bone cracking when her husband moves slightly, wakes her up.

This has had its consequences, of the most direct that now she is more sullen, any subject that is against the way she thinks, alters her and she feels offended and bursts as she never did, of course, she does not sleep.

The only time she feels calm is when she has scissors in her hand, outlining designs in her clients' hair. She has a beauty salon where she attends to her clients in a VIP manner, all of them are fixed and every month they go to her to accommodate them and while she talks to them frugally or while she listens to the nonsense that they come to tell, Ava only nods and makes a surprised face when she corresponds, she makes the gesture of indignation when she touches and laughs if she touches to laugh, but in her mind, it is not there, at least not right now, that she thinks about everything that happens.

What goes through her mind is that she has always been an instrument of others. When she was little, she grew up next to an overprotective mother who imposed what she didn't put on her daughter, so that she would do what she thought was right. As a first mistake, she put her in the best dance academy, she wanted her to be a dancer as she could not be. Ava hates dancing because she was forced to do steps, for more bad luck the teachers who touched her had no pedagogy, they treated her badly and looked down on her because she seemed to have two left feet, she was the worst in the class and they used her as an example of what not to do.

This was damaging her self-esteem, she felt she was useless, clumsy as they told her.

When her mother gave up on the subject of the dance, not without first telling her that she was a klutz, a fool for missing a golden opportunity, that she wished she had had that chance, that it is not possible that she does not value the dance if it is so beautiful and one more string of insults that made Ava feel like a rat for a long time. She felt bad, but she just didn't feel complete in doing so.

While she was thinking about this she was cutting a woman who was doing nothing but talking about her husband, who seemed to be stuck in the maid's bed, who was a 19-year-old Mexican woman with tanned skin and full lips who called Mr. Fred with a sensual and apparently innocent voice and Mr. Fred seemed to have everything removed and many hormones activated because he had the woman indignant. Ava thinks that the first clumsy one is her for putting a woman half her age in the same house and with all those attributes, obviously, the man was melting for her.

At night, at home, she talks with her husband about home issues and frugal work for both of them, when they are relaxed enough, he starts caressing her in those areas where he looks for her when he wants to make love to her. They start the sex ritual and know each other by heart for having done it so many times. She fakes the orgasm so that everything ends faster and her husband falls asleep a few minutes after finishing. Ava didn't sleep all night.

The next day, while she was cutting a man's hair, neither of them were talking and Ava was thinking about her childhood and passing to adolescence, when her mother, disappointed by her daughter who was useless, decided that she would study medicine when she was the right age and it was a very common topic at the table and they told the family on Sundays when they visited. Such was the fact that Ava would be a doctor that her cousins called her by the title: Dr. Ava. Obviously, she did not want to study that career, it made her blood run out, and seeing viscera made her dizzy, she would not be able to put stitches on even a cut finger. Less could she operate or be everything her mother said.

At the age of thirteen or fourteen, in a rebellious way, Ava began to date a 25-year-old man, the threats her mother made to her were worthless, not even the beatings, everything was solved when her father, who was another puppet of her mother, reluctantly went to talk to her boyfriend, she doesn't know what he told her, but her older boyfriend left her without explanation. Now, as an adult, she deduces that she was offered prison if she continued to be corrupted by the girl and so all this love ended before it had begun.

A couple of years later she had to go to medical school, which for her luck her mother moved heaven and earth and got her a place and thus began one of the worst stages of her life. It was two semesters where he had to endure boring classes and where he felt the same as when he was in dance classes. Of course, it was not his thing, and his mother emphasized that he was useless, that he had had all the dreams that she could not materialize and he despised them, that he would pay dearly for that. Ava didn't even complain about it, there was no remedy, her mother didn't see another point of view other than her own.

One day a classmate told her to go to her house, to have lunch and see if they would study the subject that they both had to defend. When they arrived, Ava had an epiphany. Before she was the mother of her friend, a woman who had a young girl and was doing her hair, in her own home. Ava felt in her hands a tickle that was the desire to take those tools and start cutting hair, it was what she liked the most.

She told her mother that night and her response was more contempt, that this was a job for wage-earners, for low-life employees who cut hair, that anyone could cut hair, save a few lives and she had the tools to do it.

Ava's frustration was growing and what she did was to sneak every opportunity to go to her friend's house, see her mother, and sneak in ideas.

Soon the desire to go increased when she met her friend's brother, who worked in the New York subway and would soon become her boyfriend and end up being her husband.

Ava was not a woman who gave problems on purpose, worse when she had to, she had no mercy, so when she decided to go with her boyfriend and fulfill her dreams, she gave her mother the coup d'état, announced that she was leaving home with her suitcase in hand, to college she never returned and without much preparation, she moved in with her boyfriend, his mother helped them settle in and taught her a lot about hairdressing.

For a few years Ava was happy, children who grew up, one for the luck of his grandmother, left with the desire of medicine and the daughter liked the dance, after all the miracle had been done to his mother. Everything could have stayed the same if it weren't for Ava's insomnia, she felt while cutting hair and remembering her life, that something had been lost along the way.

She needed to get the problem solved and go back to sleep, stop being so emotional, not treat her husband who was still in the subway badly, but he was a good man, without vices, who went from home to work and took care of her and raised some children who were happy.

One night, her husband was more loving than usual, she let him do it, she provoked him, half of the meeting was given up, but when she had the man on top of her, breathing heavily and telling her everything he said when they were having sex, Ava had her eyes nailed to the ceiling, she knew what was going on, it was totally clear to her now. The wrong step she took was with her husband, that man who showed up when she needed him but she used it as an escape. Her husband is about to end, her movements are becoming more rhythmic, she has become clearer with each step, she has never really loved her husband.

The man ends, she is clear now. Ava is not a woman who gives problems, but when it is time to give coups, she gives them with all the weapons, so that there is no opportunity to useless defenses.

The Husband

Every time Elizabeth wakes up, which is often at night, she puts her hand on the pillow next to her, it is empty, cold. Look at the cell phone, it's half-past two in the morning. Her husband hasn't arrived. She falls asleep, but soon after she wakes up, two forty-five, absent.

So she goes on every five to ten minutes, at 3:30 a.m. she knows she will not sleep more, gets up from her bed, walks silently through the house, expecting that the children do not wake up, arrives at the beginning of the stairs and goes down with the hope that being down she will see her husband sleeping on the sofa, but no, the house is alone, just a cold breeze coming through the window that was not closed during the night and hits her face, she feels the cold caress and a light scratch on her throat. She gets warmer and goes to close it.

She goes to the kitchen and pours a glass of water, pours two spoonfuls of sugar, stirs it, and drinks the water. She sat down in the dining room to drink a second glass of water and wait. She wasn't willing to take it anymore. She was sick of this situation.

It was recognized that she had been in that relationship for a few years by a couple who had started cheating on her since she was young when they were dating. A colleague from her job, an intern, passed by her then-boyfriend's bachelor bed. Shortly after the honeymoon, she found out that he was with another woman, this time it was also another coworker. And for years, in separate spurts of two years of fidelity with a

41

discovered infidelity, Elizabeth was tearing herself apart missing her husband a little more, feeling less of a woman because of the deceptions she was suffering.

Every time she went through these deceptions, she would stand in front of the mirror and study her face, see the asymmetries she brought out herself, feel like the ugliest woman in the world, and then her face would turn red before she would start crying and see her deformed face crying its eyes out.

She had already lost count of the number of times she had cried in front of the mirror, although she did not lose count of the deceptions discovered by her husband, the intern, the cleaning lady, the old schoolmate, the one who contacted her on Facebook and the neighbor who had been smiling at her since they moved in, Not to mention the one-night stands he was getting around and it's not confirmed, but a 17-year-old Latina who since seeing him wanted something with him and her husband's morbidness had no qualms and broke the law about that young woman's body.

Many suspicions, infinity, strange messages that seem encrypted, openly sexual messages, photos. Her husband seemed to have no qualms about hiding his affair.

The most recent one he didn't mind hiding, because he was clearly showing off with the woman anywhere, it all started when he had a company meeting, that day Elizabeth went, it was a gala night, everyone would be dressed up in a suit, be at the party and do networking to generate profits for the company. There, right next to her, the woman on duty appeared, a blonde with long legs, a thin waist, a fine face, and full lips, with a voice that sounded like a whisper and catlike eyes that looked sensually.

Her husband went crazy, didn't stop looking for him to talk and try to get his attention, even though Elizabeth on more than one occasion took his arm and pinched it so that he would at least respect her while he was present.

That day something happened that she doesn't forget, the woman in question had a smell of a perfume that was very similar to jasmine, a sweet touch, an expensive perfume, and the smell would come back to her some time later, when she found it on one of her husband's shirts just as he was washing it and discovered it because that shirt had some hair that was just the same color as that woman's.

There wasn't much more proof to look for, that night her husband arrived he attacked her and it was no use because the man did little to hide it and contrary to what she expected, he started seeing her more often, with past lovers, she saw him once in a while, once a week, but this one, was every night, the man arrived, with no smell of alcohol and with that smell of perfume that she already knew, and hated.

Shouting, hitting, insults, it wasn't worth anything, the man would stay on ice, looking at her with a disguised gesture of annoyance for seeing his wife at that hour of the morning fighting, she would leave, she would lock herself in by knocking down the door and the man would sleep on the couch.

The next day, when she was preparing breakfast, she felt her husband's fresh hands surrounding her belly, her mouth approaching her neck, the smell of soap and freshly bathed skin flooding her. He knew that one of her fetishes was to feel the freshly bathed man and he used it against her.

He would come close, would start whispering words to him, asking his forgiveness, and they would talk for a while about the evil he was doing, that he could not be unfaithful, that children, that the holy marriage. Sometimes they even made love and Elizabeth's surrender was between intense and bitter, she would reach an orgasm that she enjoyed very much but when it was over she would sink into a deep sadness.

That night, after they reconciled and he promised he would leave the woman, he would arrive late again, with an orgasmic face and the same smell, with all the evidence of having arrived from the arms of that woman.

After the reconciliation the morning before Elizabeth sat down in the dining room to wait for her husband, she had discovered on the collar of one of his shirts some lips, red, that had been marked by the woman's lipstick. Elizabeth insulted her out loud. She was alone in the house.

—Not even for a decent lipstick you have, bitch. —She said.

She washed the cloth in a rage, to top it off it didn't come off easily, it looked like a paste, Elizabeth's desire was to take scissors and cut the cloth, the side where her mouth was. But she rubbed it until it came out

44

90%. She would leave that shirt there, waiting to show it to her husband.

When she discovered that kiss from her lover, her husband had only been gone a short time and not sixty minutes had passed since she had reached orgasm in his arms, which for about five minutes had been immensely happy and then had plunged into depression.

All-day she wandered around the house, looking for memories and wondering if this time spent with your faggot would have been worth it because since the engagement he seemed not to want her, she was always on some adventure and she knew, she was sure, that there were many undiscovered love affairs. Her husband was hiding better and better every day and the sporadic lovers could never discover them, only the ones that she took hold of emotionally and lowered her security defenses. When the man fell in love he didn't care what his wife thought.

Elizabeth was tired of being the fool who pretended she was not hurt by the lovers, the mocking and the cheating, she wanted a real chance, she wanted to be loved by a man who had eyes only for her, so tonight she had given her the last chance and in bed, the dream was gone, He kept looking at his watch from time to time and in the end, in certainty, he had at that moment and discovered that it was something he had kept for a long time, he got up, went to the dining room, with enough sugar water to keep his mind cool and prepared to wait.

It was already four o'clock in the morning and Elizabeth feared that the man would not arrive, her greatest fear was that he would decide to sleep through the night, something she had never done with any lover, taking that step would be the definitive thing for him to leave, but not, at four and five o'clock in the morning, she heard the car parking in the garage, through the door leading to the kitchen, a few minutes later she felt the man open softly, trying to make the least noise, she passed, in the darkness, closed, Elizabeth could see him because she was already used to the darkness.

The man was surprised when he turned on the light and his wife was sitting there, waiting. He tried to go and say hello to her as if it were half past six in the evening and he was coming back from the office. Elizabeth stood up, in her hand, she had a gun that was kept for emergencies in the safety deposit box, she pointed it at him, holding it with both hands, she looked at her husband, the man who had conquered her heart and whom she loved more than anyone else, after her children, he was the most important.

—You pick up your things and go back to that bitch.

—Love, let's talk, I don't know what you're talking about.

Elizabeth's index finger embraced the trigger and warned that this was the last warning, if she didn't listen to reason things would be different and she was serious.

Emergency Room

Abigail wakes up on one of the unused gurneys at the back of the hospital, where hardly anyone goes, where sneaky lovers escape into a hole of the day to indulge in the honeys of pleasure.

She wakes up from a shock as her someone would have called her abruptly. Every time she woke up it was like that since her dream had become fragile. She was a nurse and had been sent to the emergency room for a month. The crudest part of the job at the hospital, because they were running all night, this facility she was in was close to one of the most dangerous ghettos in the Bronx, what came in every night were people who were wounded, beaten, shot and one who came in dying with several arrows shot from crossbows.

The ones that Abigail feared the most were injured children, the worst cases were when Christmas approached and they began to play with fireworks bought on the black market. Children who appeared with mutilated hands, with their faces marked by some burn that would damage them for the rest of their lives.

She didn't like being in this area, she preferred it when she was assigned a floor because there she would have to attend to patients with whom bonds were created, then if Mrs. Dorothy from 35 who had cancer, but every day smiled as if she enjoyed every extra minute and said that every moment she had was a gift and she couldn't complain, because it didn't make sense.

Or the sullen veteran from 42nd Street would yell at the nurses, but he would look at Abigail with a strange expression and let her be cared for.

So little by little, they created a relationship with everyone and she liked that, because except for a few blue alerts when an unemployed person entered and for a few moments the doctors tried to save his life, everything went well or if they didn't take him to the corresponding unit, but otherwise, under normal circumstances, everything went well, without setbacks and she liked that, everyone liked that, working in the Emergency Room was like being condemned to clean the pipes, sent to the redoubt where they had to spend nights of stress saving lives, even varying at the same time.

Abigail drags her feet for the bath, she has already slept the half-hour that she does every night, it will be until 24 hours from now that she can sleep again, she sees her face in the mirror, and she has huge dark circles under her eyes and greenish skin, what a bad look. You wash a little, brush, and apply light make-up, so you walk to work, peace and war are separated by a door. Where she walks everything is silent, you can hear whispers in the distance, when she opens the swinging door she will come to life with adrenaline. So it happens, as soon as he opens she sees a nurse passing by holding a bottle of serum and carrying it while a stretcher carrying a man complaining and soaked in blood is dragged along, her companions enter and leave other rooms, doctors she sees every night shouting names of medicines.

Abigail stays a few seconds watching all the movement, in that process between the calm and the storm, accepting that she has to be one more running, every second count, doing what she can to save a life.

She hears fingers snapping near her ear.

—Are you a visitor? —The owner of the fingers, a short woman with big eyes and a bad temper, asks the head emergency doctor, who is running around, helping out where she can and helping the doctors and nurses get around to work. Logan is her last name.

—Sorry, doctor, I'm coming in. I was on my break.

—Good for you that you're on break. —Would you like to know how much time I have here?

Abigail nods her head, provoking her boss' anger, Logan shouldn't be bothered.

Patient with left shoulder injury, bleeds out.

Says a man dragging a young boy in a wheelchair.

—Did you hear? —Logan asks and immediately answers, "Quickly save that life you're paid to sleep here.

He mumbles a bad word and goes on his way. Now that Abigail is on paper, she starts a short jog to the patient who is coming in the opposite direction.

She begins the routine interrogation, pains, how it happened, what she came in contact with.

Abigail helps him get on a gurney and removes his shirt with scissors, starts cleaning and preparing to see how

49

the wound is, and give the report to the doctor to treat when it appears.

The wounded man is a fourteen-year-old boy who climbed a tree and the branch broke, he fell and his shoulder was buried in a tube that was there. Luckily it only went through the flesh, a few more centimeters and he wouldn't be counting it.

The next patient was a woman, she came in with a bleed, she was eight weeks pregnant, after confirming she had lost the baby, Abigail helped her prepare for a cleanse and a curettage. I'm sure she treated her well because when she left the area where she was to wait for the orderlies, the woman said thank you with her face bathed in tears.

The night is still young, she has to attend to more patients, choose one of the many who enter without stopping in the emergency room. She had to apply a painkiller to a man who arrived with a stitch in his kidney, apparently suffering from stones, three injured on motorcycles, one with a broken leg, the other with an arm, and all three with scratches on all sides and second and third-degree burns.

It's 4 a.m. The patients never stop arriving. The Emergency Room never sleeps, only at dawn, between 7 and 9 in the morning, there is a brief pause to begin the frenetic rhythm of the day, where the emergencies are different, people with severe pain, work and domestic accidents, but the night is one of death, blood, and pain.

One night a patient arrived who was totally different from everyone else. He had no injuries of any kind, the gesture was not one of pain, he looked calm, but he was brought in a wheelchair. When Abigail noticed him, he already had his eyes on her. She was a bit startled because she looked at him with great confidence, but also with pleasure, that face seemed kind to her, not to mention that he was nice. A very handsome man.

—"Take care of this patient," said John, who was looking for patients in the waiting room.

—What's wrong with him?

—I don't know, but he asked urgently to be seen. He's been there for hours.

Abigail asks the mystery man to come with her, puts him on a stretcher, and begins to question him.

—What are the symptoms? —She asks him as she inserts the blood pressure monitor and confirms that her blood pressure is fine.

—"A slight pain here," he says, pointing to the groin.

—Has he had appendicitis surgery?

—When I was a child, yes, but it's not that pain, I remember that pain, it's different.

—Is it very intense?

—Not very.

—I don't understand then, why did you come in the middle of the night to the emergency room if the pain is mild? You could have left it for the day with your doctor.

—Yes, I understand your hesitation, I happen to be dying tonight.

Abigail was silent for a moment, analyzing the man's response, asking him if he had any other pain, if he had ingested poison or if he was being threatened with death, anything was possible.

—I have nothing of what you say, he said, —I only know that I will die tonight.

—How do you know? —I don't understand you, if you're playing a joke on me I'll call security and...

—The tarot told me.

Now if I was confused, I didn't understand anything. But something made her feel that the man was telling the truth, even though her nurse's analysis made her think he was a man with a problem in his head. Crazy people have an incredible talent for appearing credible, just as they believe their craziness, body, and verbal language feel real. But this one didn't seem so.

She questioned him some more, the man was a Spanish teacher in a rural school, lived alone, worked in the mornings, and read Agatha Christie's novels in the afternoons. He told her all this, then told her that he was going to meet a very beautiful woman in the hospital, who was suffering from insomnia and who missed love since she had lost someone special long ago.

—"I'm sorry I couldn't meet you sooner," he says with a smile.

Abigail looks at him, surprised, feeling exposed, and in her mind thinking about what would happen there. She goes to ask him more questions, but the man begins to move, shaking as if he were having an epileptic seizure, makes about ten movements and stays there, his face becomes peaceful.

Abigail sounds the alarm, quickly, and three doctors appear to take her out, ask for epinephrine, give her resuscitation, but Abigail already knows, she died.

Her death was a complete mystery, they investigated, they did an autopsy, but as much as they dismembered that poor young man they didn't get anything, it was as if the body had simply been extinguished.

The Rejected Woman

He was the perfect man, she met him at one of his jobs when they met the first time the crush was immediate, they began to talk and you could feel the connection, the desire to know each other and the taste they had. It wasn't difficult to meet for the first date and also for the first kiss to come up, which happened in the middle of that first date.

The desires of the flesh were also present, he let them appear and she also let go of some garments, but she did not allow it to happen, sex on the first date, no, Abby was a decent girl and would not allow it, no matter how much she wanted to. She was able to hold out until the third, where she accepted his fifth invitation to her house, taking advantage of her parents' absence.

The first meeting is one of those magical ones that take place between couples who seem to know each other from a past life, no matter how many people they have been with, that is the ideal one and no one surpasses it.

The connection from then on became deeper. They started dating formally, she took him to meet her parents at a Sunday dinner, he brought her back home when the parents had already returned from a trip, and both families were fond of each other. He would help with the Sunday barbecue at Abby's house and talk about cars with his father-in-law and she would talk with her mother-in-law about the church, dating issues, and even her jobs when they were visiting.

It was no surprise when the courtship was made more solid with an engagement ring he gave her that belonged to her grandmother, then her mother, and now her.

She started a job in a textile company, where she would take the administrative part, her career and he had now changed to a business where he would have to do multilevel, although the company of this service was extremely strange, he had never heard of the company. But this one promised juicy profits for him so he entered.

From the moment he entered that company, the boyfriend changed completely, he stopped being the same loving man he had always been, although he treated Abby well, it seemed that every one of his acts were fake, he felt forced to make every gesture, every word of love and even in sex, where they used to mix, Now it was a relationship where she felt used, and when it was over she didn't feel full, full of pleasure and protected by the warmth of her man's love, no, now she felt empty, with a strange depression, like when you have sex with a stranger at the disco and the next day you have a moral hangover.

She begged him a thousand times to explain what was going on, but he said everything was fine, he filled her with words of love, he spoiled her and Abby believed him, she had to do it and they returned to the tense calm where every day they were distancing themselves.

The date of the marriage was getting closer, her mother had made the preparations, they had looked for a wedding dress, the trousseau, the borrowed, stolen, blue, and everything was ready to have it that day. Her fiancé was very excited, he also said he was preparing everything.

When the marriage was one week away, he called her and asked her to come on Wednesday, three days before the wedding, to St. Simons, Georgia, because he had to tell her something. This is one of the Golden Islands, she is full of doubts and I wait anxiously and with the hope that she could recover her fiancé and return to what they were.

Those days were painfully long, because in passing her boyfriend almost didn't call her, when the day finally came she appeared in this romantic town, just where she always saw herself with her boyfriend when they went a few times in the past and there he appeared.

They hugged for a long time, more because of her, who was so happy to have him by her side, to feel him, to smell him. Finally, when they broke up he looked at her with a smile, that smile that she loved so much, and told her that they should talk.

—We must talk about something important.

—What you want, my love

—We are not getting married.

Abby's face was one of bewilderment and the beginning of a breakup that fragmented her into very small pieces.

—I don't understand what you're talking about.

—The company, which requires my work in India where it is based, I'm leaving tonight, I won't be able to marry you.

What could have been expected happened, she cried and complained and he told her that it was the best thing for her career, if when she returned everything continued, then they could get married, but the man's attitude already showed the lie, he had simply changed it for his career and that love he claimed to profess had been a farce.

Abby returned with her soul torn apart, at home she cried in dismay, for many hours, hugging her pillow, biting it, shouting insults, screaming her name.

She had suffered for love, but never for one where she was at the door of the altar, so close to the one she believed to be the love of her life, and now she would have to throw everything away, she did not understand the attitude of her fiancé, what had happened to him, how he left the wedding lying down, why he did not invite her to India, she would have followed him to the end of the world because she loved him.

Her parents tried to encourage her, but they were not lucky, every day was the same as the day before, without bathing, she went to the bathroom, saw herself in the mirror, ugly, untidy, and crying, eating reluctantly what they put in her mouth, just enough not to die of starvation. Her friends came to see her, but she didn't receive them, she just stayed in bed all day, reminiscing about what happened, feeling and wondering what she had done wrong, blaming herself, seeing scenes, words she said, messages, trying to find out what she did to lose the love of her life, so that he would end up leaving her for a company.

Some days he began to check his networks, read the messages that were said on Facebook, those of WhatsApp, interpreting his words, also his own.

Little by little, she began to feel that deep sadness, moving to mild anger, a couple of days towards herself, but then she recognized that it was towards her ex-boyfriend, she read again all the conversations and remembered the scenes that they lived, remembered her body language and felt that there were things that did not fit, that words were slipping through the cracks and were not as honest as she could have expected.

Then she began to see, to realize that she had been stupid, blind, like all women in love and that she was the only one who wanted to get married, that soon after they got engaged the changes began to take place and she had not opened her eyes to that, that her man's attitude was not the same and she had not realized it, that she seemed to use her cell phone more, details that her brain found an explanation for, but that now made sense. The man had backed down after asking for the engagement, her man had repented, he didn't want anything formal with her, and he didn't want to be imprisoned in the marriage. But she was so in love that she realized it.

The day she discovered that she was not guilty, that her love had been honest, she felt great relief, it was a strange sensation, like when you get a bullet in the head and you do not feel pain, but you feel a daze. That day she went, took a big bath and came out renewed,

58

went to bed and slept well, without nightmares, the next day she went down to eat and her parents did not say anything, but they saw the joy on their faces, their daughter came out of the abyss.

For several weeks she was around the house, did not talk much, spent her afternoons by the window, drinking chocolate, and reading, immersed in her thoughts, reflecting, and every day a little more responsive.

A month later she decided to go out, a friend invited her for a coffee and she said yes, she dressed in jeans, a simple blouse and went to see her, they talked all afternoon, her friend tried to get information from her about the breakup, but Abby was emphatic that she did not want to talk about it, so they started talking about everything, except love.

Little by little Abby returned to her life again, she found another job, the previous one was thrown out because she had left it behind, she spent several months going to work and returning home, always feeling in her mother's nest all the security she needed.

But one day, finally after so much pain, so much sorrow, Abby felt free of sadness, she could already think about her love relationship and felt neither anger, nor pain, nor sadness, she wanted neither good nor bad for her ex, she was like a simple stranger, the broken relationship was an experience, not to fall again, she was ready to return to her life, to return to her dreams and now renewed, a new version, where she learned lessons and knew how to love herself first before others over her.

One day, in a meeting of friends at the house of one of her best friends, a boy approached her, nice, with the evident intention of flirting, she opened up the options, she was ready to want something again, but always keeping her radar up, she would not go back to her first dream. Never again.

The Sailor

The sea was an extension of his body. Martin had grown up with the sea, since he was a child his father had been a sailor. When he was born, his father was at sea and met him two weeks later. Throughout his childhood, he said goodbye to his father many times while he was on the ship.

It was inevitable that Martin would end up climbing onto a boat, he did so when he was ten years old, he accompanied his father on a short half-day trip, they were going to do some shrimp fishing. The sea left him hypnotized, the immensity of the blue water, with a beautiful sky and the calm swell, creating a swaying of the boat that far from making him seasick, as happens to many beginners, lulled him and made him recognize that he was born for this, to be at sea, doing anything.

They say that we come from the sea, that the first forms of life were given there, and that later we formed ourselves, surely it was the sensation that Martin had to be able to connect in that way with the sea because he felt like he had never done it on earth, that is why at the age of fourteen he imposes himself and says that he will not study anymore, that he has clear that he wants to go into the sea, to be a sailor like his father.

This was a fight in the family because they didn't expect him to give up everything to go to sea, their desire was to have him professionally, as one always dreams of with children, with the professions one always desires, doctor, lawyer, architect and the other careers that families consider politically correct. Many were angry, some were in favor, others against, but Martin was clear about it, he wanted to be a sailor and that was it, whether the others liked it or not, he cared quite little. His father, in punishment for him to change his mind, put him to work on a boat, but a fishing boat, and one of the old ones, where he had to work hard, hoist the sails, attend to jobs on the engine, carry from one side to the other and work as a man, this for a fourteen-year-old boy could be a lot of work, But Martin, who knew that he was doing it as a punishment, so that he would back out, did not let himself be frightened and firmly endured the mistreatment and did not complain once, on the contrary, he showed himself proud and tried to do things as well as possible.

His father, seeing the young man give himself with that gallantry to everything he imposed him to do, discovered that he was passionate about this, that no matter how much war they made, even if they thought they won the battle, Martin could go to study what others wanted, he could be a professional, but he would be unhappy.

With bitterness, he accepted that the young man loved the sea and there was nothing to do to separate them, his father admitted it and from his own experience he knew that the love of the sea is not taken away by anyone. He himself declared that his son would be a sailor, if that was his wish, then go ahead. And so it was.

Martin started working hard, he did very hard jobs, he paid hazing to work on ships, but then he grew up because he was really born for this. He was good, he stood out, he was promoted from cabin boy to the first officer, and then he managed to have his own ship, he was the captain. How elegant he looked in a captain's suit, in his medium-sized ship that would cross the ocean for a couple of months.

His time on the ships forged him a slender, defined, and natural body, he who was of a thick build, by taking care of himself as a worker on the ship, it made him a man with a broad back, defined arms, and thick neck, crowned with blond hair and a wide smile, with a golden skin color that made him a very attractive man. He was aware of his beauty and that's why in every port he had a love, giving fame to the myth, women waited for him eagerly, arriving after months of absence that made the man goes from the swaying of the waves onboard the ships to the swaying of their legs.

The only thing he had, as a rule, was that this work was his life, he didn't need to be involved in love, and besides, he and the boats couldn't be separated. Nor could he be in compromise, because a woman was an anchor and would be an anchor that would not fall to the bottom of the sea, but would remain in the concrete and from there it would be difficult to set sail without suffering damage to the length.

So he fell in love with them, but his heart remained intact, some of the women who waited for him in the ports moved him more than others, sometimes tired of waiting for him, they went to the arms of another man, but when he heard that the woman was breaking up with him, he simply did not care. Many times that same night he had an-other one wrapped in his sheets, letting herself be carried away by him.

So Martin's life was exciting, he spent many weeks at sea, stopping in ports, where he drank little because he was not a man of being on land getting drunk, nor going with prostitutes, as they did much, no, he played the house, went out, met the woman on duty and spent some nights together, where this, if he had a house, filled it with gifts, made food and made love to him like never before.

When he had to return to the sea, he would say goodbye in the arms of the woman and she would bathe him in tears in the port waving a white handkerchief.

Sometimes that same night or the next he was already in another port, in other arms and between other legs repeating the ritual. Everything was majestic, and he would have continued like that unless in one of the ports, when he got off, he went to the house of a woman, a 23-year-old girl with whom he had been having a relationship for eight months. When he arrived at her house she approached him and told him that her boyfriend was there, that they could not have anything. She told him to leave, that they had been having an affair. Coincidentally, her formal boyfriend had been in Afghanistan for two years, and she, being free of her boyfriend, while he defended his country, had given herself into Martin's strong, golden arms.

The sailor was not pleased, because since he was at sea he had been thinking about the journey he would have on the body of his girlfriend, but soon recovered, went to seek his life, did not want to go to discos, or places, where they sold liquor because in these there were only women or prostitutes and if not charged, were not the most faithful that is said.

So she let the universe itself guide her, she walked away, via an immense plaza where you could see a lot of life, at first she thought it was a fair, but when she arrived she knew she was in another place, the first thing that surprised her was a strong smell of incense that shook her nose and made her sneeze, all the people seemed to be in their own way, free, people dressed in their own way, even if they were not in fashion. It wasn't one of those Comic-Con meetings, it was something different. An art center, where there were painters, poets on one side reciting, people singing.

In all that tumult, his eyes met a beautiful figure, it was a woman who had a huge brown hat with a strange cup on top. It looked like one of those Harry Potter hats but combined with an Indian touch and a witch's touch, it was strange. It was worn by a woman who was in her forties, but seemed to be the age of a teenager, she looked cheerful and when he noticed her, the woman had already seen it and was studying it.

—"You don't belong here," she said, smiling.

—Why do you say that?

The woman paused and then said

—You look too stretched out, too correct, but that skin makes you look like a man of the world, of the sea.

—I'm a sailor.

—A sailor? Well, you're not the version of a sailor I have, you're usually...

—Settled in a bar, flooded with rum and whores

The woman smiled and admitted that this was what she was trying to say, albeit in more subtle words.

The two began to talk and became friends and were strongly attracted to each other, at least that's how he felt, and he didn't want to stop talking to her. What made him most curious was that the woman was so close but so far away, she was very assertive. She showed her interest in him and that night, she let him know by making love to him as no woman had ever done before. But there are connections that go beyond what a woman or a man can or cannot do; it is when souls are truly united and know how to know each other as they deserve it.

So, the one that had looked for so much came to him, the anchor that nailed the man to the earth. She knew this as soon as she had the woman before her. They began to leave and the day Martin had to sail on the boat, he made up an excuse not to leave that day, or the next, or the next. He even gave the goods he was going to transport to a colleague of his and thus saved himself from traveling. All this marked in a way that helped the two of them to get closer together and just as when he was fourteen years old he knew that the sea was his destiny, now with little more than thirty he knew that the waves and the swaying of this woman were his new ocean. So he sold his boat, started a life on land, and didn't care what anyone said to him.

Martin was not a man of anchors unless they were those of true love.

The Sacrifice

She was a powerful woman in the community. She had land where cattle cared for and treated the land, crops that covered much of the city, and money for even the most macho men of the day to respect her.

It was 1832, at a time when women should not be in her position, but Aurore was and did not mind. She was always a submissive woman who did what her husband told her to do, but when he died in bed from a heart attack, it was her turn to assume, she would not allow the church or any other man to come and put his hand in what was rightfully his.

So this woman, who had been submissive for years, emerged and imposed her word. Everyone was surprised to see how Aurore silenced anyone who needed to be silenced, the way her word was law, and the way her slaves showed her respect. She was a just woman, she did not like to walk around the lands wielding the whip or asking Moedano, her black foreman, to whip any insurrectionist black man.

Although the times she was touched to do it, she did not have mercy. Mainly in the beginning, when the man died, the slaves believed that now they would be free or would have the power to get the lands, this was the thought of the dishonest, the honest thought that their luck would get worse, they would be sold, given away, shot, anything went through their minds.

The rebels stood before the woman, their mistress, and when she gave them an order they could not hide their laughter. Aurore was recently widowed, the comfort zone, although not pleasant, had her protected and now she had to face the same attitude of a man, something she had never done, but that seemed to be made for her.

Moedano was by the woman's side, he respected his mistress, although he also seemed to have his reservations, he had never liked having women bossing him around, not even his wife. The last one who sent him was his mother and she stayed in Africa.

But when the slave was reluctant to collaborate and even mocked, what other slaves imitated, he realized that it was now or never that he had to impose himself. He did not measure the consequences, took a step beside Moedano, took out the resolution that he always carried the belt, and shot the disobedient slave in the face at point-blank range.

—Does anyone else want to challenge his master's authority? —Said Aurore, firmly.

They all remained silent, lowered their heads, and said nothing, even Moedano extended his hand when she returned the weapon to him and he seemed scared, he did not expect it.

—I am your master and you will do as I command. I don't want any other behavior like this, because I will have to shoot them all, I wouldn't mind buying new slaves. Is it understood that I am the new mistress?

They all answered, "Yes, ma'am."

Aurore returned to the house, walking firmly, as soon as she crossed the door, she went up to her room, when she entered she closed behind her and stayed stuck to the door, shaking, her hands could not stay still. She spent the whole afternoon locked up and asking God's forgiveness for having taken a life. She knew that she was in a situation where she had seen men and her husband do it many times, or die.

Since then, Aurore's word was written in the Bible, it was respected and no one dared to refute anything. The story of the shooting of the slave ran like wildfire through the city and the attitude towards her changed, although she was a woman, they already recognized that she had between her legs some big goods, as a man and that she was even more angry than a man.

Surrounded by this story, others followed, all of them fictional, like the one where a slave did not run the errand in the five minutes he had ordered him to do so, but in fifteen minutes, which is what it took to do it, and which, armed with his tail, had ordered the other slaves to tie the man to two horses so that they could pull his head and foot until they were cut in two.

Because of this, Aurore was respected and feared and began to enjoy a life that no woman of her time could have imagined, even many men did not have her respect and position. Although Aurore was not one to go to parties or to drink tea, nor was she one to go to snobbish meetings where people came to speak ill of each other with arrogant airs. No. Only one thing was important to her, to have the money to live, to have attention with her slaves, and most important of all: to have her child safe and sound with her comforts.

69

Her little boy was only 7 years old. A sweet boy who had inherited everything from her, loving, tender, always looking for affection and very obedient, his father many times hit him and called him effeminate because he did not have that mischievous energy that he allegedly had as a child, his son had come out calmly and as he was always in his mother's arms, then he would shout to both that this boy of a man would be dressed as a woman and committing immoralities in some dark street.

Aurore didn't worry about any of that, she had seen her little one light up when she saw Claire, the Thompsons' neighbor, the farm that was a couple of kilometers away. A sweet, adorable, blonde girl who would melt away when she saw her son and he would glow when he saw her, there was childish love there.

But her father never saw that, he just reflected his own fears. Now that the woman was a widow, the boy, although he didn't say so, was happier, he could walk around the house without the fear of finding himself in some room with his father swollen with anger shouting any insult to reduce his self-esteem. Just as the woman had been transformed, he too had changed and seemed to be beginning to enjoy his true childhood.

Some time after her husband's death and being an authority in her house, when everything seemed to be going perfectly, a critical situation arose, the child seemed to fall ill from one day to the next. One morning he did not leave his room, as usual, when his mother went to see him he was pale, on the floor there was a trace of vomit and he looked very weak.

His mother looked after him that day, and saw that he was not even holding back water. After noon, he called the doctor who came to see him immediately and checked him, finding no diagnosis, he said cholera, typhus, drinking contaminated water, infections, he did not know and the woman realized that he was being erratic. This made her even more desperate, because it was no use drinking plants, chamomile, paico and even a plant that was recommended to her by one of her slaves.

The child continued to get worse and seemed to lose weight, three days into the illness, the doctor looked at her with regret and told her to prepare for the worst that a strange illness would take her child away at any moment.

At night, Aurore was at her son's bedside, placing cloths on his forehead to soothe the fever. She heard the front door knock three times. When she went downstairs to open the door, she met Moedano.

—How is your son doing, Mistress?

—Bad. The doctor said that... —he drowned out a cry and swallowed thickly, trying without much luck to stand up to his slave.

—I think I have the solution for him to heal.

Aurore's face lit up for a few seconds.

—We can help you, but there is a price.

—"I don't understand," said Aurore skeptically.

—Your child could live, if you're willing. What are you willing to do for your child?

—"Whatever," said the confident woman, looking defiantly at Moedano.

—In Africa, we have a person we ask when one of our loved ones is ill, and we would do anything for them. We all already have a score to settle with him. If we ask him now, I'm sure his son will wake up well.

—I will do it. —She said with determination.

—It's expensive. Are you willing to give your soul in exchange for your child's health?

This puzzled Aurore. Moedano realized this and explained.

—The day of her death is written, as is that of all beings on this planet. The day I die, I would not go to heaven or hell, the entity of which I speak would come to look for you. It is the change of one soul for another.

Aurore remained silent for almost a minute, thought about her son dying upstairs, and knew that she would accept; not to do so would be to start living her hell from now on, totally, she was already condemned to hell for having killed an unarmed man.

—I accept.

Moedano nodded his head and asked her to follow him. In the center of the quilombo they had a bonfire. That night, Aurore experienced things that she never imagined existed; they scratched her head with something very sharp, but in a superficial way, the blacks sang and danced and she saw shadows and entities that seemed to come from hell.

At dawn Aurore went home, exhausted, with her body aching, she entered the house afraid that all this had been a deception, but when she crossed the door she heard the wood creaking, her son was running down the stairs, happy as every morning, hungry and full of vitality, as if he had never been sick.

A couple of months later, Aurore had already forgotten everything that had happened, but she would remember it 35 years later, being at home, old, with a weak body, feeling that death was approaching. Some shadows began to creep out of the corner of her eye and when she was about to fall asleep forever, she saw a huge black shadow coming to collect her outstanding debt.

Aurore willingly gave herself to her destiny.

Concentration Camp

Run through the dark streets of the city. Already now the androids fly over the night and are looking for heat waves to find any intruder that wants to pass to paradise.

Madison has already spent a couple of hours avoiding this danger. But the machine has the clue and does not want to let her go, the system knows that there is something and would give its existence to catch her. She runs through all the dark alleys, hides among the garbage but listens in the distance to the buzzing approach, she can't stop.

In one of the alleys, she found an immense trash can that had 25% water in it, she got into that dirty water, with a bad smell, to hide the heat wave so that the android could continue its way.

She put her whole body, face-up, when the device illuminated the can, she submerged completely, the surface of the water left some waves, this was detected by the device that stayed almost a minute watching. Under the water is Madison, her eyes are open, saving the limited oxygen she has, begging for the machine to leave, otherwise, she will have to go out and they will detect her and she doesn't know what her luck will be, no one who catches will return. All women are taken somewhere they never leave.

She feels bubbles in her ears, which move and go inside, her neck seems to be closing and she has an immense desire to stick her head out and breathe. She prays for the machine to go away. When the android is about to surrender, he flies over and leaves, and she goes out and takes a breath of air, coughs a little and makes silence, tries to recover the air trying to make the least noise possible.

She listens attentively, she does not feel the android, and she seems to have been saved. She gets out of the trash can and stays there for a few seconds recovering, the water runs off and falls to the ground, she feels the cloth sticking to her body, and she feels cold bristling her back. She goes back to the hideout, she had no luck finding food and now she is five kilometers away, she has to go before the sun rises.

She takes some steps and an immense light comes on her back, she turns around, it is the android that was in the dark, watching over her. An alarm goes off and he shouts Intruder, Intruder. Madison starts running again, but she feels a strong blow all over her body, she falls and looks tied up, she has just been caught with one of those electrified nets, she was thrown by the same android, who now takes flight and carries Madison hanging as if she was a stork with the baby in her beak.

This is already another United States, although at one point at the beginning of the 21st century, women tried to assert their rights, they achieved feminist movements, in 2030 a very old Donald Trump took over the power of the United States and the first thing he did was to remove all the authoritarianism he demonstrated in his first term. He abolished many things, he censored the media, he ended the wars and some good things, but the worst thing he did was to sow an ideology where women were put in the background, first, he took away all the rights, the marketing they used was to coerce men to feel rejection and this was achieved in less than a year, they felt repulsion for women, getting them to become displaced was not so difficult. Many men opposed it and were branded as traitors and exiles.

Five years later, women were living underground, along with men, and society had been divided. On one side, with amenities, were the pro-Trump men who had places of recreation where they used women sexually, or asked them to do housewife type things, to satisfy that need they couldn't have.

And underground were all the women and some men, surviving in ghettos and going out to find food.

It was said that women or insurgents who were caught would be taken to concentration camps and others said they would be taken to places where they were executed.

Madison is one of those women from the ghettos, she was just a teenager when everything changed and she had to run with her parents underground, since then everyone went out to the earth to look for food, animals, possums and fruits and returned to the hiding places, many went out and didn't come back. This had happened with his father months before.

Many managed to escape the androids, who were the night police who went around hunting women just as the police hunted migrants on the border with Mexico. Something that no longer happened either because since the United States had changed it had also decided to expatriate many Latinos and those who were found on American soil, stepping on the country that did not belong to them, were annihilated. At first, this generated a worldwide scandal, but it kept happening that ended up being taken as normal. The coyotes lost their jobs, Latinos stopped looking for the American dream.

Madison was looking for food when she was detected, she was trying to get into a house that looked lonely, she made a noise with a piece of metal and this alerted the android that she has a supersonic ear. She started to run, found many hiding places until she found the one in the trash can, but she still ended up falling in front of the android.

She was very afraid, already feeling one more corpse, imagined that the android would fly over the sea and throw her there, tied up, to drown, a simple way to feed fish and get rid of corpses. But the machine started flying over mountains, so Madison thought they would go to an active volcano and throw it there, a simple and clean way to eliminate it, but also, after flying over several mountain lines, they found an illuminated and immense place, like a high-security prison surrounded by many mountains.

The android began to descend into an open area and carefully deposited the young woman. The net that was holding her opened like a cocoon and Madison was free. She stood up and was surrounded by many women of all ages, dressed in white clothes. They looked at her curiously, she was one of them, a newcomer.

A woman helped her to her feet, a fat woman who greeted her with great kindness.

—Hello, you can call me Adele.

77

—What is this? —Madison asked.

—It's where all of us who get caught end up.

—A prison.

—A concentration camp.

—Like the Nazis.

—Yes, only they don't put us in gas chambers but put us to work in mass production, like the Chinese, to make Trump brand products.

—"The new slavery," says one woman of color.

Some male officers showed up with long guns that weren't firearms, but were shooting electricity. When they appeared, all the women lay on the ground and waited with their heads facing the ground. Madison was the only one who did not imitate the behavior. This cost her dearly because one of the officers gave her an electric shock that knocked her down. A metal mirror. She was already wearing the same clothes as the other inmates.

I was only wearing that suit, downstairs I had no underwear, and it was a zippered panty, similar to orange prisoners' clothes.

At five o'clock in the morning, two policemen came in with guns and forced her out, pushing her around, repelling her as if she were disgusted just because she was a woman. They took her to a bathroom and forced her to undress so that she could bathe; she had five minutes to empty her guts, take a bath, and come out brushed.

Although the policeman who pushed her was looking at her in disgust, Madison felt the lascivious look on her face.

She bathed and rested in seven minutes, came out, and was hit by the policeman with the other end of the gun.

—I told you five minutes, bitch.

Madison was assigned to the area where they made Trump bags, which went out in droves and never ended. Now they handled the men's line, and very little of the women, of course, those women from the top leaders who did get accepted. But what stood out the most were men's products. Although Madison knew that in other areas they were making masses for women, all to send to Europe and other countries where they bought Trump's merchandise.

On the second night, the cell door opened, and the woman who had taken her in on the first day, Adele, came in with two policemen in the back.

—Hello, little one, how are you?

—Good. What's going on?

—You see, the day you arrived, I welcomed you, I informed you of where you were and, well, I allowed you to bathe alone in the bathroom without the eyes of others. All that cannot be given for free. I helped you. Now you owe me a debt.

—"I didn't ask you for anything," said Madison, who was already finding out where the conversation was going.

—I'm sorry. You do it, or my friends..., so as not to make a long story out of it, you could wake up tomorrow with a sudden heart attack, you'd be charcoal by breakfast time.

—What do you want? —She asked, gritting her teeth.

—"Half your food ration," said the woman.

Madison had no choice but to accept. She was looking at a woman who had power in that place. From the next day on, each time they served the food, a different woman, all from Adele's group, would walk by with an empty container and serve themselves her food, many times more than half.

Madison didn't have the blood to be anyone's bitch, so she planned to hit her, to kill Adele, although this was a bit difficult, since there were cameras all over the place, not a single-blind spot, even the bathroom had cameras, the toilets, any place was monitored, androids went around the premises from time to time and the officers were armed and always on the defensive.

For some reason, this woman could control part of this system.

She investigated where the men who were arrested were, and did not know anything. The other wing they didn't have access to was said to have men, but she was never able to check.

Madison was never able to do anything against Adele and spent five years in this camp, until forces from France and Russia united in what would be World War IV, where the United States was the target, ended

80

Trump's tyranny and the country would be free, beginning the restoration of order and equality for all.

Everything Started with a Headset

In these times it is common to see a young person glued to a cell phone. Always watching social networks, talking with friends, having video calls, living the youth. Although Mia didn't see her son doing that.

Since he was young, he had a cell phone so that they could talk when he was at school. That way she could be sure that in an emergency the little one would take out the device and call. He was never addicted to nets, nor was he ever glued to the phone unless it was for an important call or an online class.

Mia was in favor of not giving her son a cell phone because this was for adults. When she decided to give her son one, it was because one day they were late on the bus and it was a terrible fifteen minutes while the yellow transport was arriving and she knew that a tire had burst. No need to be alarmed. The next day she gave him a cell phone to call in an emergency. She gave it to him with all the rules, that it was a phone for emergencies, not for playing, that he could not take it out whenever he wanted, and that the device was useful, not a toy.

This was inoculated in the young man who, when he grew up and could have been allowed to play on the mobile and be in networks, did not do it, on the contrary, he decided to watch books or at most listen to a podcast or watch a documentary. He was a talented young man and Mia was proud of him.

He had become fond of a lot of cultural content. So, around his 15th birthday, he asked for headphones as a gift so that he could hear better and also study some sounds to create musical scores. Mia proudly set out to find the best for him.

She found some of Chinese brand but they promised to have everything and a very clean sound, the Chinese who sold them to her said in very bad English that if the son did not like them, he would take them to her and she would surely change them and even pay for the inconvenience. Mia found the way in which the Chinese man guaranteed her headset so convincing that she chose them.

A few days later it was the young man's birthday and he was looking forward to his presents. Each of the family members gave him their gifts, not to mention the aunt's awful socks, a games console he already had from another uncle, a couple of books he wanted from a cousin, and finally the most desired gift. The one his mother was going to give him.

He opened the special package and found a box with the headset printed in Chinese letters.

-It wasn't the brand I asked for, Mom. -said the annoyed young man.

-I know, but where I looked for them the salesman told me that you would like these better, if you don't like them tomorrow we'll go get the others.

The young man made a gesture characteristic of his age and opened them, they were a red headset opaque as the color of clotted blood, powerful, with a thick wire and a number of options. He looked for the cell phone and put the connector on it. He put the headphones on his ears, adjusted them to the size of his head, typed something into the cell phone, and opened his eyes wide when he started to listen. His face was a pleasure like his mother had never seen before.

-Are they good? -Mia asked, knowing the answer in advance.

-"They're amazing," he said, looking at the others at the table and saying, "Excuse me."

He gets up and goes to his room. After a while, he looked over to say goodbye to the others because his mother had forced him to, but it seemed that he just wanted to have the headset hugging his ears.

That night she didn't see him anymore. The next day he went downstairs, with the device on his head and the cell phone in his hands. What he had never done before was now beginning. He seemed to be out of date.

-Good morning," his mother says.

-As soon as he answered, he seemed out of it.

Mia didn't mind, she knew her son, he had always been a young man who wasn't addicted to anything, she assumed he was lost in his music, connecting and adapting, they were his first headset, what could it hurt?

The days went by and the rituals that Mia and her son had were broken, they no longer ate dinner together as they did every day, because her son always had something to do in the room. On the weekends, they didn't play scrabble like they used to because the son composed the best song ever made.

The most curious thing of all is that he always had his headset, they were an extension of his head. Although he didn't have the hostile attitudes of age, he was as out of it as any teenager who enjoys his cell phone, only in this case it was the headset that had him lost.

In the second month, Mia began to worry. One night she went to the bathroom and saw a glow under her son's door, she opened it carefully, hoping not to attract her son's attention, while opening it she regretted it, thinking she might find her son touching himself while watching some erotic video, she almost closed it, but she remembered that she had just seen the clock and it was 3:05 in the morning. Her son was on his cell phone, his eyes were wide open and he didn't seem to see the device, what he seemed to be doing was listening.

-You turn that off and go to sleep right away. -she ordered him.

Her son jumped up, didn't expect to see her there, took off his headphones, and saw his mother, detailing her. As if she had time without being there. He nodded and walked to bed. He went to bed and fell asleep immediately. Without saying a word.

Mia looked at the headset for a while, put them on a sofa in her room, and went out to sleep. Her son woke up the next day as good as new, he looked like his old self, he was talkative, he even listened with surprise to stories that Mia had told him days before and it seemed that he had never heard them.

The rest of the day they talked and shared, when night fell, the young man took the headphones again, when Mia saw that he was going to connect again she said

-With control, that I have seen you very addicted to that thing, remember that in this house we have to control the vices.

-Yes, Mom, I know.

If before the situation had been worrying, now it was worse, as soon as your son put on his headset, it was as if he had disconnected from the world, he was present but at the same time absent. She typed and stayed long enough to pay attention to what was being heard in the headset. Mia spoke to him twice and didn't utter a word, barely nodding his head as if to imply that he had heard and was now out of the way.

Mia didn't give it much thought that day, she went to sleep and the next day was a working day again. In the evenings she arrived, greeted her son, and talked a little with him, although he seemed not to be present, he was lost in that headset again. Mia did not want to think badly, she hoped it was just a stage, like so many stages that young people go through. All this changes one day when she gets a call from the school, they wanted to know if her son was okay, he hadn't been going to school for weeks, precisely since after his birthday, he was one step away from losing the whole school year.

That day Mia realizes that she is facing a real problem. She talks to her boss and goes home early, takes her car and goes on the gas to get there fast, she was full of a lot of anger and in turn, her brain was confused, the behavior was not characteristic of her son, on the way she thought it might be the fault of some woman who had seduced him, and he was floating in love and had forgotten his responsibilities.

She also thought it might be the fault of drugs, he was at the age to smoke pot or inject things, although this ruled out, and her son would not even go out.

All sorts of guesses went through her mind and she knew in every one of them that it was the headset that was to blame, the one that had brought out a side of her son that she did not know.

When she got home, she went in so quickly that the front door was left open. Mia shouted her son's name, got no answer, ran upstairs to the room, and there the door was ajar. Inside was her son, on the sofa, wriggling, with his feet dragging, looking lost, as if he were on drugs. She approached him, took off his headphones and the young man seemed to return, as if he had woken up.

Mia shouted at him, complaining that he had dropped out of school, that he was in a lot of trouble and would have to go to school the next day. The young man said nothing, he was dazed, it seemed that all the accusations were new to him.

Mia smelled the atmosphere and realized that he hadn't even bathed, so she sent him to clean up with the threat of a beating if he didn't go immediately.

The young man ran to the bathroom and Mia stared at the headset he still had in his hands, thought about it for a few minutes, and then put them in her ears. She felt the comfort of the foam in her ears, they were nice. As soon as she did so, it was as if she had teleported, felt a pleasure she had never experienced before, sat down where her son had been minutes before, and let herself go.

No one noticed that the connector on the hearing systems was not connected to anything. Her son's cell phone was unloaded under the pillow.

A Working Woman

She met her husband when they were just 19 years old. She fell madly in love from the first day and liked every act her husband had, filled her up, loved the man very much, and showed it to her at all times.

He seemed to be a good man, attractive, pleasant, with a gift to please everyone. He smiled with a smile of white teeth carefully cared for by his mother.

This caused Bonnie a love and adoration for this man that at the time was noticed by her parents and also by her friends. Even one of her best friends, Aby, withdrew her friendship when she noticed that Bonnie would not listen to her. She told her that she could no longer be friends with a woman who could not see beyond her nose, and that adoration of a man did not go with her.

Bonnie took it as a betrayal, when on many occasions she had heard her lovers' dislike, now she could not enjoy being in love with her. Selfish, that's what she thought. At that time she didn't give it much importance because she was in love with her partner and even more so when he went to the house and with the greatest formality in the world officially asked for her parents' hand in marriage.

Later his parents felt honored that such a beautiful woman from a good family was chosen by their son to share his life. The two were married in the eyes of God on April 19 in a small church and only with their families, this at the request of the groom, who said it was so they could have an intimate space where no one would bother them and they would be comfortable sharing only with their loved ones.

They traveled to Niagara Falls for their honeymoon, hugging and sailing in the boat where they saw the waterfall. Bonnie was thrilled, watching the couples declare a thousand and one ways and she was standing next to her new husband.

They stayed in a modest hotel, but she didn't care, because from the moment they arrived the man brought out his dominant side, something that excited her and she let herself be loved in the thousand and one ways he asked her to, as a good wife and willing, she gave in to many games she enjoyed, some even with a little pain, but it didn't matter, all to please him.

So she felt totally connected to him and on that honeymoon, one of the best moments of her life, they made the first child, who was born nine months later. During the pregnancy, the man treated her very well, indulged her every whim, spoiled her, and when the little one was born he behaved like the best father of all.

Bonnie was always by her little one's side and when her husband asked her to travel somewhere to try out business, she went, for her everything was her husband, for him whatever it took, until the end of the world, to a collapsing Chilean mine, to the Amazon to extract gold or to the bottom of a burning volcano. Together until death.

During one of those trips, she became pregnant with her second child, this time a female was born, with whom her husband broke up, she was his princess and he took her wherever he went.

He filled her with many gifts, spoiled her, and was a great father. The little girl felt lucky to have her father so attentive to her and he allowed himself to be spoiled as well.

To the outside eye, they were the typical American family, the woman with the short hair, settled in the beauty parlor that morning, the children playing happily, the husband with a cigarette in his mouth, reading the newspaper with his legs crossed, the dog jumping up and down to the rhythm of the children's games and a white railing outside with the grass finely cut.

As the years passed, the couple settled in like any other, with routines, accepting the good and bad in each other, going out for walks every now and then, and dealing with the growth of the two children who soon arrived at high school and were considering college. They had been living in the same house for years, and it wasn't long before the couple would be alone when the young men took a trip to college. The first one to leave was the boy and soon after the daughter, both good, obedient children who were happy to leave their mother's womb to live their lives.

Some time after the children leave and the couple lives alone in that house that seems to be getting bigger than ever. One day the husband seems to be sick, he started with a severe fracture that followed with a vomit of blood that forced them to go to the hospital. He had stomach cancer that had spread to his liver. A few months later the man died, becoming one of the family men who would be forgotten in the next generation.

Bonnie was left alone and felt helpless, as a child would feel when abandoned by his mother in a terminal. Not knowing where to go. She spends a few days in this grief of being left without her husband, who for many years was the love of her life.

Being a widow, she began to think about her past years, and a desire was born to get to work on something that would give her life meaning. So she enters one of those pyramid-shaped companies, where she starts at the top and takes advantage of it to recover those friends from the past, to call them to go for a coffee and offer them to enter the business.

Bonnie looks like another one, because she looks confident, she looks independent, her children are surprised because that woman had not always been the shadow of their father. Now she was someone who without a commitment to children or a husband was doing something for herself after so many years.

She quickly grows within the company and her income becomes juicy, although what she is least interested in is money, what she likes is to feel alive, active, achieving things that she never could in her life.

One afternoon, while she was at home drinking coffee from her husband's cup, she put out her hand and let go of the cup. Even with coffee in it, it fell and shattered, spilling the liquid all over the floor. She had just realized something: she hated her husband.

She hated him from the first moment they were married, when she began to notice that the man was never as loving as she dreamed. They went on their honeymoon to the place where he should have asked her to marry him and not in his car, taking the ring out of her pocket and performing the ritual with annoyance.

Nor should he have subjected her to his first sexual encounter to acts that are asked of a prostitute, so many new things in so few days in a fleabag motel.

She couldn't stand so many trips, so many changes in her life and in the end when they settle down it's in a house that he liked but she hated, neither could he ever be in the places that she wanted so much, she always had to go to his side and her dreams were forgotten for years.

When he became ill she should have been by his side, until he finally took his last breath and with this, the chains he had put on her for twenty years were over, she was free and happier than ever.

That day she didn't even dry the coffee that later became a sticky stain, nor did she pick up the broken cup. She went into the bedroom, took out her husband's clothes, made a pile of them, and set fire to them in the garage, along with all the things that were meaningful to the man. She didn't want to have anything of his in the house, she just wanted to forget him, something difficult, but it was clear that the chains had been broken forever, she was free as ever.

From then on Bonnie recovered her lost youth, she looked less years old than she really was and was a working woman who enjoyed every day. Soon she was one of the most admired in the company where she worked and she climbed to high levels. She was there until the day she died, where dozens of people fired her and remembered her for many years.

She did have a meaningful life.

Finding Love

Callie was looking for love since she was young. She was always a romantic woman. When she first entered school, she was enthralled with the boy she liked so much and when they went out to play she gave him a kiss, he was another boy just like her. The little boy was frightened, as it usually happens with men when a woman shows interest

That's how it happened to her throughout her life. When she was in school, she made out with some boys who took her for an easy woman, because she was always looking forward to getting a real boyfriend.

Even as a teenager the boys were looking for her because they hoped to get a second base with her. When Callie liked a boy, she would show it by giving him some kisses and let his hands go through spaces that she had not had before. Her breasts were then pawed by many and some more daring boys, who, in the midst of the passion, would put their hands in her crotch, but there her modesty would jump up and down.

Time went by and finally when she was about to graduate, the field marshal put his eye on her, he was the man she had always wanted, in the middle of the party they had, drunk both of them, he took her to one of the rooms and after a few morbid words he stripped her and they had quick sex that was far from what a girl expects for her first time, painful, without subtlety and with the bitter taste that remains when it is a meaningless sex. Callie, far from feeling the pleasure she expected, was depressed and went home, where she cried for a whole day without clearly understanding what was going on.

Every person is born with a desire that they want to achieve no matter what, for some reason Callie was always in love, she could never be described as a slut because she was not, she never cheated on anyone and her mind only ran with totally innocent thoughts where she wanted a man to tell her that he loved her and to go with her like all those soap opera stars that had taken so many sighs from her.

But this type of love did not end up arriving, she did not have that boy she wanted, who sighed with her, who wrote her love poems, who sang songs to her with an off-key voice, who looked at her and even begged her for a little love. Callie was very dreamy, always thinking of all kinds of scenes where the boys looked at her with their little eyes of a slaughtered sheep and asked her for a kiss and she would beg, but in the end, she would jump to hug and kiss them.

She had a subscription to wedding magazines and she knew all the variety of models, the best in the market and what the princess of such a country had worn for her wedding and she imagined herself in that dress with her beautiful dress next to it and on the altar, receiving God's blessing.

But it did not happen, that desperation to find love had made her a victim of comments, the neighborhood whore, that whoever came to seduce her could have her and in part it was true, what many ignored was that she was opening her heart every time she received one of these men and hoping to be reciprocated just as she did with them.

There is no evil that is there causing harm that does not end up generating a scale in the person. This is what happened to Callie, who got tired of having those kinds of men in her life who only showed up to put her to bed, and when they satisfied their desire, they didn't return her calls. Then she began to feel a resentment towards men that became more aggressive, more painful every day. Even when a man came with lewd intentions, she looked at him with disgust and did not accept. She had her weak days where she would allow someone to seduce her and go to bed with him, but then she would throw him out herself before giving way to harm.

She would sigh in her loneliness, wishing she could have the opportunity to be loved, she would deny her pain because the loved one was not there, but she would not allow anyone to notice, even in the neighborhood people would comment that now she was not seen with anyone, some men would say that they had tried to seduce her but without luck and this was a joke because if a man was not able to take Callie to bed, it was very bad to seduce.

But they soon realized that she was another one, that she didn't want to continue being the talk of the town, that she couldn't take another insult from some woman who called her a slut because she had slept with her boyfriend or worse, her husband. But Callie hadn't even noticed that the man was engaged, for her the man who appeared with seductive intentions, was because he was free and wanted something serious.

You may think she had a screw loose, but no, she was an extremely intelligent, hard-working, professional woman and had even known how to knead money, only that she found it a bit difficult to understand the sharp or dark sides of love, that not everything was like soap operas and that love was far from what you saw in Disney cartoons.

So, from being an easy woman to pick up, who with four sentences would go with the guy, she had now become an airtight woman who saw any man's approach as a threat.

Morgan was a long-time colleague of Callie's, and he witnessed her hanging out with several men from the company and then greeting each other as if nothing had happened. She never looked at Morgan with any other intentions, and he watched her in silence without even paying her a compliment, even though he was taken with her from the first day he saw her.

He liked the woman very much, she was attractive, smiling, kind, and intelligent and he felt a strong attraction as he had never felt with any woman, the only thing he felt like a weight, was that she behaved like a slut and seemed to have no self-respect that stopped his advances to seduce her.

Although he felt relief when he heard in the corridors that she was rejecting men and that now she wanted to adopt an attitude of dignity, as if they did not know her.

Morgan felt a slight burning when he heard these derogatory comments. One day, when he feels up to the task, he approaches Callie and they talk about work, the weather, and anything else. He looks for a way to ask her out. When he told her, the woman changed her attitude and looked down on him.

—I could have expected it from anyone, but you, Morgan? What a disappointment.

Then she walked away and left him there, bewildered and not understanding what had happened.

A few weeks passed and again Morgan had the opportunity to talk to her, after setting the mood he told her.

—I don't know what you understood the other day, I would never want to hurt you, I didn't mean to offend you.

—I didn't mean to offend you. I'm sure you do, like everyone here, you have a fixation on me, if you want to empty your testicles, go to a brothel, use your hand, I'm nobody's toy.

Morgan was going to try to explain himself, but the woman came out at a fast pace and left him with the word in his mouth.

Some time later he approached her and went to the point, with sincerity.

—I've liked you ever since you went out with your friends, ever since I saw everyone saying bad things about you that I tried not to hear, I've always liked you. I never dared to say anything to you because I wasn't the Callie I wanted, despite the strong attraction I had for you. But now, where everyone comments that you reject them, that you walk alone, in search of yourself, I am even more attracted to you and my intentions to go out with you is to get to know you better, not to get you into bed, I care about you, what you are, not your body. I like you, Callie.

The woman looked at him, moved, but without saying anything, she put her hand on his shoulder and left.

That night at home, Callie's head was a whirlwind, she thought about all that Morgan had told her and that he seemed to be what she had always looked for, she thought about him and she had never seen him as a prospect, but she thought that he was not bad, that she could accept a coffee from him, talk to him, get to know him a little.

The next day, she was the one who looked for him and told him to have a coffee.

When they left work they had a coffee far from the stress of the office and began to feel that they had many things in common and that they were comfortable, little by little they got to know each other better and formed a stable relationship, an idyllic love as Callie had always wanted. Love had finally found her, when she had stopped looking for it as a desperate person.

The Breakthrough of Perfection

She's looking at the ceiling, that white, polished ceiling that her husband arranged so carefully. Now he is an orphan, as is she, the new widow.

Since she died her dream has not been the same, but how can it be if for thirty years you slept with the same man by your side. The love of life, with whom you first shared a bed. When they were young and fiery, they gave themselves up and felt their skins; when love calmed down to give way to a more leisurely relationship; when they went to bed angry, and even when they had that lover with whom they almost left the house and when they made up, they lived a sort of second passion.

The bodies deteriorated in bed, fatter, with less smooth skin, wrinkles, and aches. It is known that at some moment one of them will leave this world, but this is as hard as saying goodbye to the mother, one knows that someday she will die, but to accept that she is not the woman full of life and now she is an old woman, it is very difficult to accept that that side of the bed will be empty forever.

How love hurts. Even if you live with a couple for many years, finally the sunset comes where one leaves and the other ends up crying about the departure of this one or giving thanks because he left, everything depends on how it was.

In this case, Celia, our protagonist, misses her husband very much, she feels that the bed is itching, that she is hot and that she is immersed in an ocean of mattress, that the bed is too big for her.

She gets up, puts on her slippers, feels them too hot on her feet, and walks barefoot, feels the ice cream on her soles, and is relieved by it because she is hot.

She goes to the closet, opens the door and sees her husband's side, there are finely arranged all the suits she wore during her life as a married man and businessman, clothes made to measure, perfection, the man was perfect, a whole picture, a real gentleman, he fell in love with her the old-fashioned way and never failed except for the time of the crisis when he fell in love with another woman, but he was always a man who respected her, who never spoke to her in a bad tone and even his anger was in style.

Years as manager of his own company, he knew how to educate his children with discipline, with tenacity and made them good people who also managed to reach the highest levels of quality. In front of her, she had the remains of a man as few are born in this world, and how she missed him, how she felt the weight of absence.

She noticed this every morning when she served an extra cup of coffee and then remembered that her husband was not there, she threw the cup in the sink and cursed her luck. She said that she should have died first, not her husband, although later she thought about how she would have taken it and surely she would have fallen into a depression and suffered more, because that is what Celia had, that although she suffered, she was brave, she was tough and did not break down so easily,

102

her husband, although he was brave, on an emotional level sometimes broke down before her, and this blow surely she would not have endured.

Two weeks after her husband's death there was a knock at her door. When she opened it was a young man with a FedEx T-shirt holding a box in his name that was already paid for.

Celia signed for it and took the box, saw that the sender was her husband, was very surprised to see her husband's name on it, opened the package with trembling hands and hurled some insults at the shipping company for closing the packages with such dedication.

When she finally removed the wrapping she had a small wooden box in front of her that had paper inside. She opened it and put her hand to her mouth, because she almost started to cry. He began to pass the papers one by one, everyone knew them, they were already worn out by the years, but they were those, his love letters, many of those she wrote for him, wrappings of knick-knacks, photos of when they were young with signatures behind each other. The many details that the two of them gave each other when they were engaged and in the spring of their marriage, each one of the details, was such a dedication with which he had kept her, that many did not even remember them as much as he remembered them. When she finished checking everything, she found a new sheet of paper, which looked recent, had her husband's shaky handwriting, written in black pen.

Dear and beloved Celia, I am starting to write these letters with a lot of pain, because I know that if you read them it is because I am already dead.

Life was so cruel that it took me first than you and now you are alone. I'm sure you are surprised by this box you received, but let me tell you that all this time I have kept it with the love I have had for you since day one and I hope that on the other side of life I have them too or that I live like a loop the wonderful love story you were.

You are the best thing I had in life, you who gave me the other wonderful gift, our children, I love you very much, and I hope from the other side to protect you and watch over your dream.

I love you. Don't forget to drink the chamomile water with plenty of Stevia so you can sleep and don't suffer from insomnia, even more so now that you're upset about my death, which I know you, when you're stressed out you don't sleep.

All-day long she read the letter and reviewed every detail the husband had put in it, the story of a love narrated in letters and details of decades of marriage. Everything or had saved what man keeps those memories?

This was not the only thing, because a week and a half later they played at her place again, this time it was a florist company that brought her an immense bouquet full of pink flowers and coves, they made the arrangement as if it was a swan and her husband was the sender.

When she unfolded the leaf, it said in his handwriting:

Happy anniversary, my beautiful, such a day as there is we got married and it was the moment I was happiest in life. I hope that at this moment you have by your side this arrangement of flowers made just as I asked, the pink flowers as you always liked, the coves you loved so much and the swan that was the symbol of our love, and that united us forever since we were young, when we knew that swans once in a couple, is for all life

Not even death will be able to untie the love I feel for you and my demonstrations of this eternally for you. I miss you, I don't know where I am now, but I know that from where I am, I miss you.

Celia felt bad, guilty, because she had forgotten the anniversary, she was going to fold the sheet, but she realized that in a fold there was a message for her.

PS. I know that at this moment you will feel guilty because you didn't remember our anniversary you never did, it was the joke of our love, I sometimes forgot it. Right now you are forgiven because it should not be difficult to deal with my death, so do not feel guilt about it, on the contrary, feel happiness that today in our day, you have before you those beautiful flowers that will remind you how much I love you.

Celia smiled bitterly and knew that her husband knew her more than anyone else, even after his death.

During the following days she took care of protecting the flowers so they would not die so soon, when her death was inevitable she took a cove and a rose and kept it folded with the letter, to keep that beautiful

105

bouquet in mind, she also took a photograph so she could contemplate it as much as she wanted.

For several weeks her husband did not manifest himself, but she knew that soon she would have another detail. Her birthday was coming up. That day, at noon, while the children were at home, sharing their birthday with her, there was a knock at the door, when she opened it, some mariachis started singing with a man with a beautiful voice. When the song ended, the mariachi said that it was a present from her husband who from beyond wished her a happy birthday.

It was a bittersweet serenade that had one more detail at the end. The only woman in the mariachi band came up to her, took off her huge hat, and handed her a letter with a sealed envelope.

—This is what your husband leaves you, he sends you to say that he will love you forever and he is waiting for you on the other side.

She gave her a kiss on the cheek. Celia felt her cold lips and was left with the feeling that she had left lipstick on her skin.

With her index finger she caressed the hard texture of the sealing wax, she always took pleasure in these stamps. They looked so elegant. She opened the letter with trembling hands and took out the sheet, unfolded it, and began to read.

Happy birthday my wife.

By now the mariachis must have already sung, I looked for the best one of all. One that you always praised me,

106

I hope they sang as they suggested in their advertisements.

Love, this is the last letter I will send you, I think the previous ones and these left a painful taste and I do not want you to suffer, enough with my absence.

The purpose of these letters was that you could keep in mind that it doesn't matter anything, from where I am I love you and I protect you, just as I had in mind to give you all the details that you have received, I also took care of every detail, you will never lack anything, not even me, because from here I protect you.

The letters I gave you and the details were to remind you of the beauty of our marriage, so that you will remember the beauty and not get caught up in my death.

Finish enjoying what you have left of life, that when God calls you, here I will be waiting for you on the other side.

Always yours...

Her older son sat down next to her and stroked her back

—What's going on, Mom? —he asked, worried.

—Nothing, son, everything is fine, only even if one does not want it, the end of perfection always comes.

The Burden of All

From: Cadence <CadenceM@gumal.com>

Date: Mon, 7 February 20 at 7:32

Hello friend. How I miss you, I'm missing a lot to talk with you and to be able to connect to tell you all the changes I'm suffering now. In the last email, I told you how I'm doing with my pregnancy. Uff, the last few months were terrible, I was throwing up every day, I had cravings and a mood where I hated Roger all the time.

I feel immensely happy, seeing him there, that little thing that came out of me, that sees me with those little eyes full of so much innocence, that smiles at me and loves me, that gurgles out words and I want him to say mommy.

That little being has changed my life and you can't imagine how happy I feel right now. All I need is you, to be able to listen to you, to be able to tell you so much, and for you to tell me that I am a romantic to die for and that at some time it is telling you that being a mother is a cross.

I don't believe how this beautiful little thing could be a cross. Although I confess that ten minutes ago I felt my hand full of something slimy, it was the baby's poo, no matter how much soap and water I poured on it, the smell doesn't seem to go away.

Write, my friend, that sometimes you forget about the poor beings, of course, as you are in Paris, seducing Frenchmen and drinking wine, since we don't even write to the poor newborn. Ungrateful.

With love... Cadence.

From: Cadence <CadenceM@gumal.com>

Date: Mon, February 27 at 9:30

Hello friend. I've had a rough month, the baby made green poop and was also spending sleepless nights. He didn't sleep at all, so the next day I had huge dark circles under my eyes and he was sleeping divinely.

Not to mention how my tits are on fire from all that baby sucks and you're going to tell me that he's a little boy, that he's going to hurt me if he doesn't even have any teeth, well he does, it's like he's going to rip my nipple off.

I've also spent a few days where I get very depressed, I don't know why. Although I'm better now, I'm getting better, the pediatrician told me that my depression was part of the hormones.

We are complicated. I liked the photos you sent me from Paris, send others.

I miss you.

From: Cadence <CadenceM@gumal.com>

Date: Mon, 12 March at 15:30

Hello friend. Thank you for what you say about the baby, yes, he is beautiful, at least he doesn't look like his dad who looks like a coconut, he is handsome my prince, I feel like eating him with kisses.

I'll tell you a secret, sometimes I see him sleeping, he has several hours like that and I miss him, I wake him up gently and when he starts crying I lull him to sleep and devour him with kisses.

Although surely this is what all mothers do.

With love.

Cadence.

Merry Christmas, my friend, Santa Claus is coming home tonight, the boy still doesn't understand about it, but we bought him a big cuddly toy of a cat, which he loves. Besides clothes and details to make him happy.

This year of so many challenges and so many things is already closing, Jeff who went to Afghanistan, the baby who has taught me so many things, work, Roger, in short, everything we have suffered and enjoyed.

But today is not the day to be thinking about those things, but to enjoy and be happy for the times to come. I am honored to have you as a friend and again, it is another Christmas without your presence. Without you by my side.

I miss you, I wish you a Merry Christmas. Don't get drunk, as always.

Merry Christmas.

From: Cadence <CadenceM@gumal.com>

Date: Mon, March 20 at 8:10

Friend, the prince started to walk, we all got excited here, he put on his two little feet, shaking, with a huge laugh because he knew what a feat he was doing and then he took some quick steps. Running and arriving at my side, we all applauded him.

Now he's walking all over the place, holding on to what he can, like someone who can't swim and is inside a pool.

Here is the video we recorded for you to see.

From: Cadence <CadenceM@gumal.com>

Date: Mon, July 16 at 4:32

This boy is already over two years old, and since he absorbs that boy, he runs all over the house, but of course, since he learned to say some words, he starts screaming like crazy.

Sometimes I ask him to calm down because there comes a point when I can't stand his screaming. Does that make me a bad mother?

I love my son, but some days he overflows. I feel that I need a break, I go into the bathroom, and soon after he shows up there, knocking on the door with his little hand, he doesn't want anything, just to be pampered or to show me something. He already starts to show spoiled behavior.

That child promises, he has character.

PS. About what you told me, yes, your boyfriend is an idiot, you shouldn't have let him do that to you. In your shoes, I would leave him to learn.

From: Cadence <CadenceM@gumal.com>

Date: Mon, May 05 at 3:21

The little one is already in school, he looked beautiful in his academy clothes, incredible that he is already three years old. Not long ago I had him in my arms and he fit in my forearm, small and beautiful. Today he is a little man who says No to everything, and before that, he used to say "why" every time I explained something to him.

Being a mother is incredible, but some days I despair of not being able to do many things or that the child is not as idyllic as it appears in the diaper ads. But I love my child. I love him with my soul. He is my life.

When will you have your child?

Look, you're going to run out of those eggs.

From: Cadence <CadenceM@gumal.com>

Date: Mon, 5 February at 7:32

My child is already 7 years old, how these creatures grow without one realizing it. The truth is that I am surprised with this child who is now a little man and many times I have to get hard in order to face him. He has his character.

A few weeks ago I spanked him because he said a bad word to me, I promised him that the other one would be in his mouth. He has to learn to respect his mother.

It has been difficult, this motherhood, because you start thinking sometimes, children are the best thing in life, but then you sacrifice so much, you leave dreams to be fulfilled, I think that when I am older I will be able to take out of the drawer of memories everything that I could not do now.

From: Cadence <CadenceM@gumal.com>

Date: Mon, 14 June at 9:26

I know what it's like to have a teenager. It is terrible. Today he told me to go fuck myself, yes, like that. That child that I gave birth to, in pain, broke me in half. He told me to go to hell and he did it with rage, with rejection. As if he hated me.

Could it be that he hates me?

That's not all, he has days with a bad attitude, Roger tells me that it's part of the age and that he has his character, that adolescence is difficult, but what mother is prepared for a son to say something as horrible as that. I don't think any. I can't stand so much pain and I can't handle this.

I'm in my day, so everything affects me more, it hurts and I feel that my son doesn't love me. Could it be that he doesn't love me anymore?

We don't even talk anymore, I remember when he was eight years old, less than five years ago, when we were at the table, sitting, talking about everyone as if we were best friends, now? At this moment I am his number one enemy, that child no longer cares about me. To him, I am just a simple general who asks him to do chores around the house and to do his homework. That makes me an enemy.

As soon as I begin my adolescence, what years await me. This child is going to kill me.

117

From: Cadence <CadenceM@gumal.com>

Date: Mon, 31 August at 10:38

I am writing to you worried, my dear friend. I was putting away the boy's underwear and I found a joint, a big joint about six inches long, to take a few puffs.

I remembered our youth when we smoked our own joints, but I never imagined finding my son doing the same thing, I guess it's the law of life. But now, thinking like a mother, I have my alarms on, because I imagine my boy with an injection machine and his face missing because he injected meth.

This afternoon when he arrives I will talk to him, to tell him that he has to stop smoking, for sure it will be a difficult fight, because he is getting worse every day.

The saddest thing is that my husband doesn't want to support me, it reminds me that we both smoked and we did worse. It's true, it's karma, but I'm sorry, I won't be quiet when I can read the letter to my son so he can stop thinking about doing drugs and ruining his life.

It's already 16 years of this young man, there are two years left and he will be an adult, how I wish I had that little baby, that the worst thing that could happen to him was that he would have a shitty ass. Nothing else.

Being a mother is a gift of life, but also a punishment.

Are you never going to give birth? Not anymore, you married that rich Frenchman who didn't want kids. You were really smart.

Cadence.

My Lover

I don't remember when we met, I just know that one day we were talking like two acquaintances who want to know each other more.

It happened on Facebook, he appeared on my account and greeted me one day, then he told me something else and then we talked constantly, little by little the hints came out and then we met in person, in a shopping center that was some distance away from each other and that was quite lonely. There we gave each other some delicious kisses, that I do remember, our first kiss, sitting on a bench in the mall, we looked to the sides where no one could see us and we devoured each other, I felt the hot blood of that brown woman, because her tongue ran down the mine and moved like a snake inside my mouth.

That day my hormones were raging, I wanted to take her to a hotel. Although she didn't want to.

From that day to the second date nothing was missing, we met in another part of the city, took a cab and there we went talking about everything a little bit, as if we were going to a business meeting and not to a hotel to get to know each other naked.

When we entered the hotel, we chose a themed room with a round bed and a dome that showed the stars at night. With a bathtub on top where we could get in.

She is the most beautiful woman I have ever loved. So in our first meeting I was very nervous, she kissed me, and started to undress me little by little, she went

119

through parts of my body that I don't want to name here, but that you will have no trouble imagining. Her tongue was not only good at kissing, her expertise made my fear go away. So that day we did it there, but for some reason, I had a resistance that made me repeat with her six times, as if I were a teenager, we were in the bathtub, in bed many times, on a strange piece of furniture and in a position that we loved, me on the edge of the bed and her on her back carrying the rhythm of everything while we looked at ourselves in the mirror.

That day time seemed to be very short, although I must confess that several times when I was enjoying myself more, the guilt wrapped me up, even in one of those I visualized my son running towards me, greeting me, and my wife also looking at me from afar, but they found me like this, naked making love to this woman and seeing the pleasure in my eyes and my body pearly with sweat.

My lover made me forget that feeling of guilt, massaging my back, and giving me an orgasm where I didn't have one.

We continued to see each other, that day and many others, where we met in any corner and went through each other's bodies as we had learned to know it. Something that makes me feel guilty is that when I go through it I feel something that I have never felt with another woman, I have the pleasure as it does not happen with others and I could make love to her all night long, without any problem.

When I think about it, the guilt corrodes me, it is so much that although we both feel so comfortable, I also feel bad and I distance myself from her, the first time I blocked her from the networks and the cell phone, she called me from many other numbers and at the end, full of anger I insulted her and told her to leave me alone.

I don't understand how she can love me if she knows that she is the lover, that when we are having sex in bed at two o'clock in the afternoon, at night I will go to bed with my wife, with my son, in my home. I would not be able to fall in love with a married woman who at night could be having sex with another man. I would not be able to stand it.

For a few months, I managed to keep that woman away, writing to me about false accounts, discovering her by the way she talked, and blocking her again. Always fearing that my wife would realize the betrayal.

One day, I started to miss it, I regretted having blocked it and I unblocked it. She seemed to realize that, because soon after that, the friendship passed to me and I accepted it. We started talking as if nothing had happened and a couple of days later she asked me why I had left.

I explained to her and she told me that I didn't have to worry, that she knew her position, that she didn't ask me for anything, just that I loved her. How hard is it to be a lover? The temptation won me over and we met again, we did not say why, but the meeting was near a hotel and she arrived in a gray cotton dress that looked beautiful, after talking a little we went to the hotel and there I found her beautiful body with a lingerie that had a bow, to open it as a gift. I unwrapped my gift and enjoyed it to the last drop.

That day I was not at all to blame, the scoundrel made me enjoy it like never before, we rolled around in that bed and moaned.

I didn't say, with her there was no worry of pregnancy, she had two children and was sterilized, so we could do it without fear, she would never have children again.

We were dating for a few months and she was afraid I wouldn't leave her again. Sometimes, when she writes to me and I don't answer her soon, she writes to me with more alarm, that if something happens, that if I'm okay. Then I show up and explain to her why I didn't respond and she seems to come back to life. I feel a little guilty about that, because it hurts me that she is so afraid. I don't want her to feel that I don't love her, because I do, I love her and I wish I could be with her longer.

Our dates are always for sex, just once we met and went to a park that is a few hundred meters from a madhouse, it is a place where no one goes, there we went to a small waterfall where we took off our shoes and felt the water on our feet, fresh, divine. We kissed and felt so much that day that we were dying to go to a hotel. But we didn't, we wanted to repeat that encounter, but the next time we met again we locked ourselves in a hotel to make love. That day was phenomenal. She gave herself away like she hadn't for a long time and we tried so many positions and in so many ways that we were exhausted. When we finished we went to a painting conference that was being given at the Museum of Fine Arts, where as the happiest couple in the world we sat down to enjoy the words of the speaker, smiling mischievously, because nobody knew that a few hours earlier we were moaning with pleasure and asking for more. If you ask me, I think that was the best day of all for us.

Although shortly after I did it again, it happened to me when my wife behaved well with me, I felt that I did not deserve so much love and I sent my lover away again, there as the woman did not understand, I insulted her, I said terrible things, I made her angry and then we fought. Not to speak for months.

Many nights before going to sleep I thought about her and how wonderful it would be to have her in bed right now, but then I would fall asleep and never dream about her.

A year later, when I thought I had forgotten her, we made a date, she gave Me Like to a picture and I told her, so we began to talk and we met again in a sleazy motel where we enjoyed ourselves, but we felt that a connector was missing, that things were not the same, she made me notice it, but we did not go into it in-depth, but were entertained at the moment.

One day, we had a little friction and she spoke to me in a way that was like a balloon bursting, I was totally disappointed, I stopped feeling anything for her and the supposed love I had for her is over, now, if she lives or dies I don't care, although every now and then I log in with a fake account to her Facebook and check her photos and think about how she will be.

Sometimes I imagine I'll walk in and find pictures of her and a formal couple and feel a bitter pill choking me. I wouldn't want her to become a bad taste, it's not for me, because I have my wife, but I wouldn't want it to be for anyone else.

Since I left her, I sleep better, the guilt does not corrode me, before, during our time as lovers I could not sleep, and I woke up. Sometimes in the middle of the night, I would wish for her and calm them down myself, but I never spoke to her again.

Although, a few hours ago I liked a picture of me, one from 9 years ago. I know it's her, it's her way of acting. I'm thinking of talking to her, or maybe not. Although an afternoon full of fire with the fire of her body would do this being good.

The Young Man

She was tired of having to put up with everything her husband wanted to do to her, she had to face every day all sorts of scorn and meet her husband and the smell of cheap, prostitute-like perfume, she said, because no other woman would wear something of such bad quality and much less mess with a married man.

For many years she has put up with a man who has not valued her. She has never lacked anything, she has money, she has comforts at home and she travels whenever she wants. Her husband holds a major political office, in addition to having multi-million dollar businesses. They live in the most exclusive area of the city and with 360-degree panoramic views.

That's why Chastity can't stay. She has everything a woman could want, plus she was born in a poor neighborhood and went through hardships before positioning herself as the wife of a businessman, who then used her as a trophy. When she met him, she was just a young girl, and the man was already his age, 10 years different to be exact. She lacked nothing, she was beautiful, with an angelic face, with a mischievous look. But the man who would be her future husband filled her with details, sent her to have surgery, put her breasts, made her increase her buttocks a little bit and operated her nose and other little details, all this with trips, luxuries and the latest in fashion and technology. The young lady from the neighborhood became the lady of the important businessman, who later entered politics.

Few know Chastity's past, for when her husband was known throughout the United States and the world, she was already his mistress. But men, when they have power, want more, so after having his wife safe and giving her everything she wanted, she started looking for other women, mostly young girls.

Chastity fought, made scenes, and took out those neighborhood roots that characterized her, all in order to prove that she was the lady and the others were the bitches. It didn't work, a man with power is arrogant and blind. What moves him is his ego and that is what hurts him most when he is hurt.

That's why she decides to start a plan. She opens a Facebook account where she puts her best picture and starts following a lot of guys. The first few days she talks to several of them and gets nowhere, just talking about typical nonsense that is talked about in networks, little by little she starts to flirt better, she flirts with some guys, but cuts them off when they send her a picture of their member without asking for it. She feels disgusted by this vulgar act. Those romances are behind her and those details of the gentlemen are now so frugal.

Finally, she manages to find a very good-looking young man. He is 22 years old, studying music, white, with pink lips, finely combed hair, easy smile, friendly, with a rich verb, and with a wide culture. His name is Kevin, they start talking and Chastity is captivated by being surrounded by such a gentlemanly man. Besides, at that age, he is very influential and allows himself to be manipulated.

Every night, from her bed, with her silk pajamas and her expensive perfume, alone as always, she began to talk to the man. He was already there, attentive to talk, the hours began to go by and without realizing it, and they were talking at two o'clock in the morning. One night at almost three o'clock, both said they felt a strong attraction. Chastity recognized this, she liked the man, but her intentions with him were different, they were different plans, revenge was what nourished this relationship.

In the chat, she was waiting for a proposal from him.

—Let's meet.

She didn't know what to say, because the photo she had posted was one of those traps, where they showed and didn't show, a profile that didn't allow anyone to guess it was her, but which did show that they were talking to a very beautiful woman.

One night where her husband told her he was going to a business meeting, which she knew was the phrase he used when he wasn't coming back until the next day, Chastity dressed up and met Kevin at the entrance of a shopping mall. She asked him to get in the car, not to meet her outside, because she hadn't confessed to him, but she was a public figure.

That night she put on a red signature dress, and subtly put on makeup, perfume, and her long light brown hair fell down her back. When she parked at the meeting place, Kevin was already there. He, who sensed that she was an important woman, was careful to dress in a suit that didn't fit him but didn't make him look bad either.

The young man entered the car naturally and was surprised for a few seconds, he didn't expect to meet the person inside.

—Is something wrong? —asked Chastity, who was beginning to feel uncomfortable.

—I didn't expect...

—What?

—No, it's nothing bad. When you told me you were an older woman, I imagined a more... mature, older woman, but you're... you're very beautiful. You leave me speechless. You are extremely beautiful, Chastity.

—You're not far behind. You are very beautiful.

They both smiled, she started the car and they hit the road, she didn't say where they were going, but the plan was to go to a retirement home they had outside the city, it was a place her husband never went to, however, when she arrived she stayed a few feet away, confirming that her husband wasn't there with some woman. When she saw no movement, she took out the remote control, opened the garage and they went in.

—What are we going to do here?

—It's a house we have for special moments.

—Wow.

—We'll be very quiet here. I have some wine that you are going to love and we can listen to music, do you want to?

—As long as it's with you, anything.

They get out of the car and go into the house. It was a luxury house, one of those escape houses that have a view of the city and that even though they never visit it, they keep the elegance that only the rich know how to put in the houses.

They talked for a while, but between the two there was already chemistry, they let it emerge at the second glass, when the mouths met and the breaths began to become choppy. She put her cup aside and caressed his face. Kevin felt his hand wet from the perspiration from the cup. He caressed her back and both of them relaxed and stripped off their clothes.

Chastity drowned out several small cries of pleasure that night, as she felt the youth of that man on her, who seemed to feel the most fortunate to be traveling with a woman he said was the most beautiful of all. When they were over she was very happy. It had been a long time since anyone had made love to her, only sex and reluctantly. She already knew that her husband had stopped loving her and had her like a vase.

Today, she remembered all of her femininity and from that night on, the malevolent plan she had to take revenge on her husband, to see if he would wake up and try to get his wife back. But the plans changed, now they started a clandestine relationship where they met at every opportunity to frolic and little by little Chastity also began to fall in love with that young man. Soon, she began to help him pay for his things, like his college, clothes, personal payments, and money to use as he wanted.

She had fallen in love, she had to admit it, and he seemed to feel the same way. This retirement home had become the love nest and now they began to see each other not only at night, but also during the day, the best thing is that they lived in danger, which is what makes everything more exciting.

Chastity began to plan the masterstroke, she asked Kevin for six months to escape, then she began to move capital, a lot of money, she would not leave empty-handed. She placed a few million in accounts that could not be violated by her husband, in tax havens. After a few months, she had enough money to escape and not work another day in her life.

One morning Chastity's husband arrived at the house, as he often did, smelling of a lover and liquor. When he entered, he lay down on the bed and didn't even notice, six hours later when he woke up with a stitch in his head and exhausted, he shouted his wife's name but she never showed up. He became suspicious when he saw the empty closet, there was little left of her in the house. From there he began to investigate, he asked intelligence to look into it and it was not difficult to find Kevin, the conversations and the first date, at which point the connection via Facebook was paused, the husband already knew who Chastity had left with, he followed the bread crumbs and saw that zeros were missing from the account, he continued to snoop around and found out that she had left the country. By the time he came to find out, his wife was already in someone else's bed enjoying the money she had taken with her for retirement.

Neither all the power this man had, nor the political connections, nor his wounded ego were able to find the woman. Somewhere in the world that for security reasons does not reveal itself, Chastity and Kevin enjoy love and money, gilding themselves in the sun and loving each other like no other.

Sometimes happy endings do exist.

Welcome to America

Finally, the boat seemed to see land in the distance. At first, it looked like a small piece of land that showed that on the other side there was hope and fortune, then it looked better, and you could see that there was life in that piece of land, on one side you began to see the figure of a woman with a big robe and a dagger pointing to the sky. Then you would know that it was the Statue of Liberty.

Welcome to America!

Shouted one of the Irish on the ship, one who had befriended one of the sailors and drank rum all the way, and his face was pink with the joy of having drunk the liquor and of arriving at his destination, as if his life was resolved when he got off.

It was the 1920s and a ship full of undocumented Irish were arriving on American soil to get a chance at a decent life. There Bryony came with her family, she was an only child, her father and mother were on the boat, her grandmother had had to leave her, her mother came back from the trip crying because it was a kind of mourning, she would never see her mother alive again and the grandmother, mother had finally sent her off with a serene gaze, as if wishing that the trip would be a path of roses and joy to serve them to move forward, although in the eyes of wrinkled eyelids you could see the deep sadness caused by being separated from her family.

The ship was finally reaching land, Bryony was seasick the first two days of the trip and her guts were empty as soon as they were full, both her father and mother were distressed, but the captain with a laugh told her that she was a newcomer at sea, that she would soon get used to it, the truth is that she was not the only one seasick, half the ship was vomiting on deck, but on the third day practically everyone was used to it.

When they stepped ashore, they were given their cloth bags and stayed there, in the port, looking around, looking for something to do. An officer ordered them to approach a kind of module, where they had a scribe taking data. Each one gave their name and this was changed to a more American name and so they entered the United States officially.

Bryony's father went through his pockets when he was already in town and found some crumpled bills, he didn't have enough money to cover his expenses. He said they barely had enough money to stay in some boarding house.

They were recommended an old hotel at the end of a blind street, and Bryony was disappointed to find that ugly room, moth-flooded wood, a bed that smelled like it had never been washed, and windows that looked dark because they hit a brick wall. The only window overlooking the street was a place where a man repaired cars.

Bryony didn't sleep that night, she hadn't told her parents, but since they had left Ireland it had been difficult for her to sleep. Now, in that new world, she felt the smells of that flophouse hitting her nostrils. She smelled of urine, stale sweaty sheets, and old wood. All this made her nose itchy and she wanted to sneeze. She was not the only one, because her mother, always silent, obedient, sneezed all night long and when Bryony looked at her, she gave her a smile like "everything is fine".

The twelve-year-old doesn't understand it very well, but they spent several nights there, even though they couldn't afford more than one night. The next day, her mother went out for a couple of hours and when she came back she was happy, with a huge bag of bread and juice for the three of them, although her father didn't eat, because he went out to "see what he could get". For the rest of the day, he did not return and Bryony was able to share with her mother and be a little more at ease without the man's authority.

That night her father returned with rosy cheeks and happy, singing Irish songs. Bryony saw her mother whispering things to him, in reproach, and the man far from being angry said to her in a waiting and cheerful voice.

—Stop scolding me woman, I'm celebrating, I've got a job, tomorrow I start.

And so it was, the next day the man left very early, looking bad because it seemed his head was going to explode, but he put on his work clothes and after crossing the door he left whistling. Her mother told her that he had gotten a job in a sawmill, he had to move wood from one side to the other, chop, unload trucks, whatever came out and also the hardest job, it was Irish, the Irish have to pay for the arrival in the United

States, if they want the American dream they have to draw blood from the soul to get it.

That boarding house would be the house of the three for a few months, and Bryony's mother was beginning to get tired, because many nights the little one heard how the wife was complaining to the husband that they had to leave, that they could not continue sleeping badly. Since her arrival in America, Bryony slept on several blankets and had her travel bag as a pillow. She didn't sleep much, so being on the floor or in bed didn't matter to her. But apparently, her mother was uncomfortable seeing her in that condition.

The fights became so intense that some nights Bryony would pretend to be asleep so she wouldn't hear the soothing breaths and body movements that ended with some strange sound from her mother or a guttural groan from her father. Bryony was very sad when that happened because she imagined her father hurting her mother, although the next day she saw her mother happy, bright.

Years later she would understand what was going on there.

A few months after his arrival, he announced with much fanfare that he was going to live in a house, a complete house for everyone, that's how it was, it was an apartment in an old building that was not far from the boarding house.

Her mother, shortly after arriving, began to feel strange discomforts, headaches, dizziness, and a great deal of hunger. She hadn't wanted to announce anything, but the prominent belly gave her away, she was pregnant.

Bryony was disconcerted and for several days she didn't know how to handle this feeling, in a short time she wouldn't be the child of the house, but there would be a new member, another mouth to feed. Not to mention the house they were in, which had two rooms, her parents' and hers, she would soon have to share. Her reign in those four walls had been short-lived.

Her father celebrated the arrival of the pregnancy and said a phrase Bryony would never forget:

Let's hope it's a boy now.

For some nights Bryony felt guilty about being born a woman, then she felt the haze that maybe her father didn't love her as he should have because she was a girl. This hurt her.

A few months later her mother said she was in severe pain, her father was gone and Bryony had to carry her mother and follow her orders, take a small bag and walk beside her, while the woman nailed her nails to her shoulders. They walked for ten blocks, at a slow pace, sometimes the woman breathed a sigh of relief and walked faster. Finally, they arrived at a hospital and had to wait for two hours until the woman finally left through a doorway into a restricted corridor.

Twelve hours would pass before Bryony heard from her mother, who was another child. She had been born well, weighed 4,200 kilos and her name was Abby, the little sister had arrived.

Her father finally showed up after it was all over and Bryony noticed his happy face looking through the glass at the little girl.

—The boy was not born, but another doll arrived, as beautiful as my first daughter.

After he told her this, he passed his rough hand across her face, in a loving fatherly gesture.

Bryony felt like the luckiest girl in the world. Years later she would understand that it is difficult to understand her parents at that age, with so many commitments, with so many burdens, it is difficult to cope with the burdens of being in a new world, in a place with so many complications and at the same time be a loving father who reminds his children that they are loved.

Bryony started sharing a room in the house at a few months old, which now smelled of baby powder, poopy diapers, and cologne.

The house seemed to light up with the arrival of the new baby, every day there was something new with him, and his father also seemed to be doing well at work, because apparently, they improved his contract, he would earn more, now that he had a bigger family and they could have more luxuries. For one Christmas he arrived with a huge radio that was the company at night so he could entertain himself. They listened to family radio soaps and the news.

That radio would be the same one that would tell the war times, the war stories, and the events that would come in the next lustrums.

Today many generations have followed Bryony, remember her as a loving grandmother with many stories of her arrival in America, some descendants amassed fortunes, others not so much, but she was part of that Irish wave that today makes up the nearly ten million American citizens.

An Ocean in Between

Love has no borders, countries invented imaginary lines in their geographies, but people all the same, except for the ID card that does not differentiate. An act as sublime as love knows it and that is why it manifests itself all the time, as can be seen in the following story.

Two people met in a chat room, he said HELLO, so, in capital letters and she responded in small letters, so they began to know each other and gradually agreed that they liked each other despite the fact that both had very different cultures, and differed in many things, except that they were human beings and felt the same.

Elliot lived in the United States, in the city of San Diego, he was a student of foreign trade, he was 24 years old, he was a gangly young man, skinny, with big glasses and a huge nose, in spite of this description, he was not so ugly, his happy, kind, always positive personality transformed his attitude into someone nice that he attracted in spite of being ugly.

In the United States, he had had a few girlfriends, but because he was so in love, he quickly overwhelmed them and they felt they couldn't continue in that relationship or they might drown.

That's why after a few months or weeks of dating, she would leave him, crying in the corners until a new woman appeared and he would fall in love with her a few days later.

In one of these periods he met his new girlfriend, with whom, although they were not in the same country, they felt a strong attraction and understood each other well.

Internet relationships have a strange good taste that makes you want to stay connected, it's an adrenaline rush of not having the person present, but at the same time, being able to have her so close, just a moment after a message, even though she's on the other side of the world.

The two started with a greeting, with the indifference that starts a conversation in any open chat, but little by little they began to talk about generalities and it seemed that the letters flowed from both sides and soon one asked the other if he had a way they could connect on the outside, a social network, she gave him the email to look for her on Facebook, he did and now they were connected.

There, he began to review her photos and learn more about her personality. He went to information to see if she was in a relationship and breathed a sigh of relief when she announced herself as single.

He saw that she was a very beautiful woman, with her cinnamon color, her black eyes, and her tender and innocent look. Her bushy eyebrows looked like the roof of her eyes that were the lanterns of the beautiful mouth that illuminated the entire face. She was very beautiful, Elliot deduced that at the first moment.

She, Dana, lived in New Delhi, a 14-hour flight from New York, on the other side of the world, in various time zones and many different cultures. She spoke perfect English and he loved getting to know Dana's rich culture. When she saw the HELLO, she responded with the same courtesy she had responded to the other seven guys who were stalking her in the chat room.

But Elliot seemed so nice, that for some reason she did not understand she ignored the other windows and started chatting only with him, then they went to Facebook from where he had a better conversation, of course, she saw some photos and with regret, she realized that he was not the gringo as she imagined him and as she has seen in the movies, but he was not so bad after all.

So, every day they start talking. When one of them wakes up one leaves a message for the other. At six in the evening, Elliot said good morning to Dana, who was just getting up in New Delhi. She wished him good night after he had breakfast. What they agreed on was that they would each get up early in their country so that they could spend some time with each other in the evening so that they could talk a little and deal with the fact that while one was earning his day, the other was sleeping on the other side of the world.

Although it may be a bit far-fetched for people to fall in love even when they are so far away, it created an affection that was more solid than anything they had ever experienced in their lives with people who were physically present.

In one conversation, the inevitable question came up: What are we? What is it that we feel?

The other said: I don't know, but I like it and I don't want to stop.

In this way the two continued to connect, talk, get to know each other a little more each day. Falling in love.

The virtual couple had the first fight one day when they made a video call, she had just gotten up, he was having dinner, and he had a huge burger in his hands.

Dana opened her eyes and watched Elliot chew with pleasure.

—What do you eat? —she asked him.

He looked at the hamburger and said what he was eating, with a tone that made it clear "can't you see?

—What is it?

Elliot responded with a full and casual mouth.

—I don't know. It's meat.

Dana changed her tone, she already knew the answer.

—Meat of what?

—Cow, I guess.

Dana opened her eyes, and with a gesture of annoyance or insult to be more exact, she hung up. Elliot called several times but no luck, no answer. No matter how many times he tried. That night he stayed up until 4 o'clock, trying to get her to answer but no luck.

They would spend several nights where he insisted on writing but she simply didn't want to write back.

It was so much insistence, so much anguish, that finally, Dana answered him. It was she who made the video call and she stayed with a serious face, looking at the camera, as if waiting for an explanation.

—I don't understand what happened. —I don't understand what happened.

—The call is not for an apology, then.

—I apologize, but first I need to know what I did wrong.

—The hamburger that filled your mouth like a beast.

—Are hamburgers forbidden in India?

—No, but cows are sacred and you called me to show me how you chewed one.

Elliot felt that some extremely valuable information came to him at this time. He remembered that Hindus did not actually kill the cows and understood that he had made the mistake of his life, that he had been a big idiot. He apologized and she forgave him, in those days full of anger she understood that although he had done her a very big offense, it was a cultural contrast that manifested itself.

They returned to the relationship as if nothing had happened, except that Elliot spoke well of the cows on one occasion, saying they were sweet and that he had seen a woman in the field petting one and this one moved affectionately as if it were a spoiled cat.

One day she said she wanted to go to the United States, but that it would be a very complex issue with her parents, he was analyzing his finances, and covering a trip to New Delhi was out of the question for

143

much of his limited income. So they were in limbo as they got to know each other in person.

The months went by in a relationship that although it felt like it was full of a feeling that it had reached the limit that all relationships could reach, the first one that began to feel the consequences was Dana, who one afternoon felt the hairs on her back stand up when she was called by her father and had a brief conversation.

That night she ignored Elliot's messages, the next day they talked, but she was no longer the same, she was distant, she didn't want to tell her boy anything, but she was afraid that he would break when he found out, it was something that sooner or later had to happen.

Elliot helped to speed it up. When he noticed that the attitude had changed, he began to stalk him and ask what was wrong. She finally told him.

—My father is a respected businessman in New Delhi, he knows many powerful and resourceful people. I am his only daughter and what happened was going to happen sooner or later, they asked for my hand, my father has come to an agreement and I am already engaged to a businessman, we have not yet met in person, but I know who he is and we have greeted each other on some occasions. In other words, this thing we have cannot go on, because I would be betraying my future husband.

Elliot had been broken up in many ways, but this was the most prominent of all. He could say that he had been abandoned because his girlfriend had been engaged for cows, goats, and land.

Dana didn't give him much of a chance to beg, when she told him everything and said it was ethical and moral to break up, he said goodbye and told her that he had been special and a few minutes later his hand with a bandage on his thumb, informed Elliot that he was blocked. They had finished.

For a few days he wandered around with his grief, but then he returned to the chat room, now hopefully looking for a woman of his own nationality or Mexican at best.

For her part, Dana, met her husband, he was not the ideal she had, but he was good to her and behaved like a good husband, they had six children and lived with the happiness that any Hindu can have.

The Unexplained Disease

Diane got sick one day. Not all at once, but the illness came to her as a slight discomfort that gradually consumed her until she ended up in a hospital.

But we began in parts. She was studying graphic design in Australia, and when she turned 18 she left Dallas for Australia to pursue a career. For some years she spent there, five to be exact, she made life, developed projects and did very well. Then, when she graduates she decides to come to the United States again, to see her family and decide what her next step would be.

Until then, she was a woman full of talent, joyful, and enterprising like no other.

Being in her city she starts to think about what she should do and opportunities arise in Australia, although it was not what she wanted, it did not fill her need for passion in her life, so she rejects it. Soon, the boyfriend she had at that moment, with whom things were not going well at all, tells her that why not analyze what it is that fills her completely, that makes her happy and that she could do all her life even for free.

For Diane, this is a cold blow because she had never asked herself this before. What it was that moved you that made you think about having the opportunity to achieve something. What her passion was. She had a real talent for many things, she liked graphic design, but it wasn't what she really wanted for her life, she expected more.

She spent several weeks reflecting on what she wanted for her life, she could hardly sleep thinking about what it was that could make her succeed, be a business that she would be in for many years.

Finally, she recognizes that she likes the world of marketing that she could develop a life there, and combined with the design she would earn very well and beyond that, it was something she liked. So she starts working, she sees the strengths and weaknesses in the business and starts to serve several clients, to give them solutions with a company that helps to boost marketing in large corporations.

Soon the clients begin to rain and she must call a friend from Australia, who was her partner for years, he had quite a few projects in the inkwell, but when he hears Diane's proposal he comes, a couple of weeks later they are starting from scratch in the city and giving everything for that business.

So far everything could be fine, but soon Diane's mother gets sick, and during a routine exam, she is found to have early-stage cancer. The operation process to extract it begins and then the chemotherapies, this coincides with the launching of a new product of the company, which generates very high stress. A lot of load, fatigue.

It is there where Diane begins to feel sick, she breaks down, the body feels sore, especially for the legs, which seem to be weaker every day and hurt. She goes to her family doctor, who leaves her in the hospital.

Here she begins a series of medical tests that keep her in bed, checking every part of her body, from her liver to possible pregnancies, cancer, hepatitis, and even yellow fever.

Everything was negative, and every morning they took blood for tests. But even though they saw the physical symptoms, they couldn't make a diagnosis. Her life seemed like a Dr. House chapter, except that after several diagnoses, House did not show up with the origin of the rare disease.

Diane's life was not the best possible right now. They say that illnesses appear because of living conditions; that was what was happening to her. Apparently, she had an illness so severe that she couldn't heal with anything.

Her boyfriend had become insecure and had started to fight over everything, and even when she was in the hospital he didn't miss an opportunity to reproach her for how lonely it felt to have a girlfriend who didn't do that. She was so vulnerable that she actually felt guilty about what was happening to her boyfriend. She asked him to forgive her, even justifying his not visiting her because he claimed that hospitals were the focus of serious illnesses and he did not want to catch them.

She did not say anything, the only thing that went through her mind was that she was to blame for her boyfriend feeling bad, but at the same time deep down there was a spark of anger because the one who should be supporting her in such a hard time was just another executioner.

The relationship was so toxic that they fought several times a day. Even in the moments when she felt the most pain, it was strange that her boyfriend asked her how she was doing. But Diane was a fool, she felt responsible for everything and she put up with it.

In addition to this, her mother was still at home, they didn't see each other because she was undergoing chemotherapy, going to the hospital could be counterproductive and cause her a major condition.

Diane feels deeply alone in this journey because her father was also dedicated to taking care of her mother while she endured the treatments, so all he did was call her, ask her if she wanted him to come, and even though she dreamed of seeing him, she told him it was okay, to continue taking care of her mother.

Her partner and friend also began to push, hoping that one day she would take back the helm of that boat where she had been mounted, so that they could make the very important launch that was frozen thanks to Diane's condition. Everyone seemed to have frozen at that moment. Everything had stopped and Diane's morale began to break down. Being in that hospital, which treated her so well, every day she felt the smells, sounds, and voices coming from every patient. She knew when it was time for the injection because she felt the smell of alcohol nearby, and then a slight groan.

She would hear devices beeping from a routine check-up. His doctor would come every morning and check her legs, and he did so with great care. Even Diane felt a little uncomfortable, but the doctor's face was very professional; he would use a small hammer to hit her in several places and ask her to tell him the degree of pain from one to ten. In the places where it hurt the most it was 7.

But although it seemed that he was being treated as it should, they did not find the evil and she did not fully understand what was happening. Neither did the doctors, although one day she began to understand everything. She realized that the hospital would not heal her. She knew this when the doctor ordered a biopsy, she of course refused and said she was leaving the hospital.

She was not discharged, but she left anyway, although she was affected by having to leave in a wheelchair, a young girl like her, full of vitality, being dragged in a chair. When she arrived home she began to feel a little better and with the passing of the days, the pain began to go away, the reunion with her father, who looked healthier than ever, with her mother who fought like a warrior and looked happy. That warmth of home first helped her get out of bed and walk despite her sore feet, her legs hurt less each day and she started working from her bed.

His partner brought him work and he was checking it out and they were preparing the whole campaign to launch the product. So, eight weeks later a very beautiful Diane was standing at the entrance of the event room, making the launch, was not quite right, but even had recorded content, made writing, and had many ideas for work that would soon be launched.

Months after the launch, when she had already broken up with her toxic boyfriend, she met a young man who was also passionate about marketing, focused, assertive, and soon broke up with her boyfriend. Each one is in their specialty and seems to be doing well. As for her mother, cancer has gone into a very good

150

remission and the prognosis is favorable, it seems that she will be able to sell cancer and the company is not bad at all, they already have several companies in the firm and they continue to arrive, the best thing of all is that Diane is doing what she is most passionate about and each day of work is not a job but a passion where she flies time away and always listens to her satisfied clients.

And about her illness, we never knew what she had because science is not capable of correctly detecting the condition of a person who is sick with stress, and in medical literature, they don't get texts where they say that invisible illnesses exist and that it is not worth the amount of blood they take out, the x-rays or the biopsies, they won't be able to find the evil, because that comes from within, just as Diane had, who upon discovering it, was healed.

Today it is a reference in marketing in the United States and last year it had a revenue of 500 million dollars. They went from two people in the company to manage 236 and the expansions and businesses continue to open every day. Diane's next goal is to get her company listed on the New York Stock Exchange.

She will achieve it, when a woman believes in herself, nothing stops her.

The Intermittence of Love

There are love stories that are made by the gods themselves, who pull the strings so that the relationships are those special ones that inspire the most beautiful verses and the most romantic stories.

The story that we are going to narrate next has as its main character Abril, who met a boy of her same age, she was older than him for some months, but he has the advantage of being more mature in many things, he has had a difficult life that has forced him to see life in a different way than many people of his age.

April, from the first moment that she connected with him, always sought to stand out, to give him the impression that she was interested in him, she talked to him, she was interested in his life and little by little she showed him the alarm that yes, she was available to be seduced to show that she was open to a relationship.

The first subtle signs didn't have much effect, but little by little he became aware of her interest and Brian realized that he liked her too. That's when the flirting started and he was surprised that he liked April so much and that she reciprocated like no other.

She would open up to show her interest in him, you could see it when they were talking and talking about sex, he would ask what he liked and she would say some things that she liked and he would let it be known that he did not like to talk about sex, but that he would surely not regret it.

Brian was a suspicious man, many people had failed him, and so for a woman to come and talk to him so openly about sex and that everything he saw seemed perfect, he was overwhelmed, where did such a perfect woman come from, the truth could not be like that. He did not deserve it, or so he thought.

Although men have the particularity of feeling the distrust, but not lose the opportunity to go to bed with the woman and this made it clear one day when he said:

—Let's meet up and go to a hotel, see what happens, let whatever fate desires happen.

So, they planned to meet and Brian took her to dinner, then he took her to a cozy, romantic hotel with a bed full of rose petals and candles, a service that was paid for and that he put there to celebrate with her.

The atmosphere was perfect for the two of them to make love with passion, both of them walking around and getting to know each other's curves, the perfections and imperfections, smelling each other, tasting each other, and getting to know each other's sounds in the games of love.

As if they were a pair of old souls, the bodies met again and enjoyed as in no moment the two had done. This made her immensely happy, she felt very much loved by him, and wanted to be the beloved of this man who did not lose any centimeter to go through her.

Brian liked it, very much, because the pleasure was immense, but he knew deep down that they were not ero sex, there was also within them a taste that

153

increased and they liked it, that no matter how expert you can be in sex there is always a connection that cannot be explained, that is not love yet, but that connects and makes those souls become one.

That's how the two of them were and soon they fell in love, although as the relationship grew and they fell more in love, Brian began to feel a lot of anxiety, at first he didn't know, but he woke up even at night with that fear stuck in his chest, he slept without understanding for sure what was happening to him, but soon, he began to be dazzled by what was happening to him, was first like a spark, like a minimal flame that told him that something was happening inside, that it could be that his base, the comfort zone that he had established and where he felt safe, was beginning to crack and he was coming to an abyss from which it might be difficult to get out, that he could stay forever in that hole, that he could return to that time where he had so many vulnerabilities.

One morning after having stayed up for several hours, he deduced that he was afraid to feel so comfortable with her. With his girlfriend, with April, having such a divine time made him feel bad, because the alarm that this woman was too perfect was going off.

That's why the first time he makes the mistake is when he goes and impulsively blocks her from the cell phone and social networks.

Poor April did not know what to do because one night they talked like the most in love in the world and the next day the man had vanished, when he went to say good morning, the profile photo of the WhatsApp was in

154

a gray face and on social networks did not appear, called him and sounded a beep, characteristic that had been blocked, in short, the man vanished. April was not a woman to stay tied, so she went immediately to take her brother's cell phone and called him, this number was not in Brian's possession, so he answered.

The man didn't know what to answer, he babbled and Abril demanded to see him right away in person and told him that she was going out to meet him, after a while, he came home.

When they were already in person he explained to her that the best thing was to leave this until here, but he didn't give her any reason and Abril wasn't going to be left with a simple breakup, where she didn't say anything, she wanted him to make it very clear what was happening to him. And in the end, after asking many questions, he ended up showing his fear and telling her that he felt insecure, that she was a very perfect woman to be real, that he couldn't speak so well, be so loving, so good a lover, she came from many gestures and seemed to be unconditional "such a perfect woman cannot exist".

She promised him that she would love him for a long time, that he was the love of her life, that nothing would end, that they were eternal, that she would not leave that relationship, and that she would not let it end, because she knew what he felt and he knew what she felt that if they could even give themselves to love right now, live, have children, whatever he wanted, because Brian was the love of her life, because they wouldn't separate for anything in the world, that's how he made it clear to them, and they started making love

155

right there, making up, and he felt safe and a fool because he had thought that way.

The social networks were restored, the number was unblocked and they started the love relationship again. All happy, in a great springtime they celebrated by going out to make love, to enjoy, to eat, to go to many places.

Love was back to normal, but Brian put it all together again, thinking about why she had been so loving in the reconciliation, then said she was insane, maybe she was a crazy person who had an obsession, like Norman Bates, the psychopath in Psycho, who would one day kill him and talk to him like his mother, while renting a room in a road hotel.

That's what he thought, full of fear, full of anguish, so the more loving she was to him, again he would behave as if he had fears, as if she were a traitor.

Then another day he didn't block her, but he was very harsh with her, he told her that they were breaking up, that no, that the explanations were too much, that the relationship was going to hell, and that goodbye. So, without anesthesia, with a lot of pain for her, she broke down, cried a lot, felt miserable because her man was leaving her and Brian took it upon himself to be such a scoundrel, to hurt her in such a brutal way that her ego was so bruised that they left each other. He did not block her from the networks, so they checked social networks, looked at photos, she sometimes left him a "like" to show that there was love. It was a very big feeling, they finally ended up talking, they ended up together.

156

Three years went by, several times he left her, they spent a couple of months apart, she cried a lot, and she was torn. With a lot of pain. At night, before going to sleep, he would hug her, kiss her, and feel that she was very far away. He was very much in love, but he wasn't able to do it. He felt the love, he felt the desire, but there was always the latent fear.

One day, April tired of that insecurity told him to go to hell, so, with that scatological word, when he showed that everything was going to end because he felt that there were failures, she threw him out, that now if they finished. He felt very sad, because he loved his beloved deeply and hoped, as was his custom, that she would beg him. But he did not admit it, he told her that he agreed, that they were ending.

The love was over forever, she thought. That weekend, she went out and accepted that person who showed her desire, they saw each other and in the midst of spite April allowed him to kiss her, but the mouth of that man did not know her love, the smell was not the same, the texture of his skin, nothing, she felt disgusted, as if she were a prostitute who kissed the client on duty, then separated from that man and left.

She was anchored to that sickly relationship of an insecure man who couldn't put on his pants, who couldn't show that there was real love, who couldn't accept being loved, an insecure man who had always been cheated on, so when someone sincere showed up he wasn't able to enjoy himself, a little man, a silly scoundrel.

On the Road

Africa Salome is an incredible woman. Since her childhood, she has stolen the gaze of men, who looked at her and felt guilty for freezing in front of a young girl who had not even entered adolescence. When she reached 15 she became a tall, slender, and extremely beautiful woman, with skin the color of her first name, Africa, a chocolate skin, soft and perfect that even the most conservative would make you sigh.

Her body also had many attributes, she was sensual, delicate, with a firm body, turgid breasts, and large round buttocks, long legs, and delicate feet, her face was delicate, with fleshy lips, big eyes, and a fine nose and small ears, her hair was a bit frizzy, but she took care of it and it fell wavy caressing her shoulders. She was beautiful, she felt beautiful, but not as beautiful as she really was. So she was erratic in her choice of love and had several lovers who did not value her and rejected those who did love her completely.

In time, she fell madly in love with several people, until finally, she tried an older man, with money, who took her to live in his luxury house, and filled her with all the pleasures that such a woman could have, after months, they were already living together, the love was intense for a while, but years later she would wake up from that lethargy, understanding that the man she was with was depriving her of so many things she had, of her desires, of her dreams, that he kindly forbade her to study music, that when she wanted to sing Cuban music she didn't let her, that when she wanted to dance she made excuses, this made her so beautiful and with so much to contribute to the world, she was deprived of it.

So little by little, she was extinguished, she became the dream of every manipulative man, a submissive woman who said yes to everything. That man had a woman who could give him so much that he was afraid and blocked her, made her little, turned her off. A man who is pitiful.

Luckily for Africa, this man finally died, one day he had a heart attack and this woman who was enjoying 37 years that seemed 27, was retired, widowed, and with a life ahead of her to enjoy and experience each of the experiences that her husband had deprived her, the first thing she did was to say goodbye, she cried to the man for several weeks. She felt that he was the love of her life, that she would be with him forever, but after a few weeks, a feeling came over her that made her feel a little guilty, the spite was combined with the feeling of freedom, she no longer wanted to be with anyone, she no longer had a chain, she could go wherever she wanted. She argued that she needed a trip, so she took a trip to the other side of the country, she looked for the Camaro that her husband loved, a colonial blue one, with two black stripes. She prepared everything for the trip, brought her credit cards, perfume, clothes, and the will to live. She got into the car, turned it on, and let the universe guide her, so, soon she was on the interstate and drove out of the city to other states, she had 49 more states to go through, to live, to know, and to forget everything.

Her first stop was in Las Vegas. That night she wore a white suit that was completely fitted to her body and made her look extremely beautiful with that sculptural body. That night she just got off with a minimal wallet and bought chips to have a few hours of fun, stayed about three hours, won, lost, smiled at her good and bad luck, and returned to the room after changing the chips she had left.

The next night she repeated the same thing in another casino, she entered, drank some cocktails, smiled at the compliments of the men many were businessmen or entrepreneurs who had a lot of money, others not so much, but all seemed to be an equal copy, younger or older of her dead husband.

She felt very feminine as she watched the men pour out their praise for her. Every night, in the hotel she looked at herself in the mirror, first in her underwear, she saw the sculpture, how the fabric stuck to her clothes and that she was indeed not an ugly woman, then, when she felt more secure about her body, she looked at herself naked, she saw every detail, the small imperfections that made her feel insecure, But then she realized that in reality, the details were minor, she was extremely beautiful, she understood that she had not been valued as she really was and that men had made her notice, and she promised herself that no man would ever come to reduce her, because she was an extremely beautiful woman who would command, who would choose and who would love as she wanted.

A week later she left Las Vegas, it was already too frugal this time, she got into her car and started a journey wherever life takes her. That's how she ended up in Utah, there she spent a few days, touring the city, both day and night, in these lands, she enjoyed Logan

160

Canyon, there she was reflecting for several days, she was enjoying all its beauties and when she felt quite at peace with herself. She started the journey to other destinations. She walked through Wyoming, Nebraska, Iowa, Indiana, Ohio, Kentucky and finally ended up in New York, where she settled permanently. The first night, after enjoying nature and behaving like a good young woman, she decided that that night she deserved to take a step she had never taken in her life. She went out to a party, arrived at a bar, pretended that she was the one who was going to be hunted, but it was she who ended up hunting, saw a man, let herself be seduced, found him handsome, and let herself be guided to where he invited her, had a passionate night where she was the one who led the pace, enjoyed it totally and when she felt satisfied, at about three o'clock in the morning, she left the hotel and went to her own, she had already accomplished it.

After having this experience on the road, where she met many people, talked, hiked, talked to hippies, smoked joints, even one night she traveled and met again with peyote, she ended up settled in this city she had never visited, she traveled all over the country to stay living in the Big Apple. She had money to choose whatever she wanted, because the man had inherited everything from her and the first thing she did was to fulfill her dream, she set up a clothing store that was near Fifth Avenue, then she started investing in art and became a businesswoman in the city, always controlling everything, the business, the conversations and even the men she went out with.

A couple of years after she was widowed and already with many businesses in full swing she decided to give herself a chance with one of her partners, a man who was a businessman too, of her same age, single and with whom she got along well, he was a free soul, who did not like to have anything imposed on him, who was very comfortable with his life and had already had his one-night stand, but they had remained in contact with the same respect, she allowed other steps to be taken, they were connecting better and they were establishing a relationship where they discovered many things in common, where Africa was not losing any of its freedom nor he, they soon got engaged and married, a few years later they had two children, who had a happy life next to a man and a woman who valued them and made them feel loved.

Africa was able to overcome the bad times, which were imposed by the canons of society, the machismo that many women suffer. But now she was free and allowed herself to be loved by a man who knew how to exploit that woman's whole body and enjoy that free soul both as a businesswoman and as an artist, because now she was beginning to try the arts of painting and was doing wonderfully.

Olivia's Apparent Insensitivity

She was a woman who had a hard look, the first person to see her turned on the alarms when she saw the body language she had. Because her face looked rigid, her frowning to the point that her eyebrows almost joined with a three-line wrinkle, as if she had a fork in that place, her eyes seemed to be flattened because she looked with expectation. Her lips were tight, her breathing was slow, like a person holding back anger, her hair was tied back in a ponytail, her words came out in a very measured way, and she was not a woman of walking giving away extra words.

She had a husband, Olver, this was an extremely nice man, the opposite of the woman, this man's words were kind, with a long smile, his eyes narrowed when he smiled at people and they all had something to do with Olver, who liked it. Throughout his life, he worked in the railroad industry, traveled all over the city as a pilot, started working from a very young age until he was quite old and retired.

Everyone in town knew Olver.

Olivia was also well-known, the woman was tolerated only by her husband, because sometimes some neighbor would show up at the house to talk, to tell some story, for example, Miss Dorothy came the other day to tell that her mother's new husband was apparently cheating on her, who arrived at dawn smelling of cheap perfume and reeking of sex.

At that moment Olivia was devouring a piece of papaya, while she listened to the young lady tell everything that was happening at home, she didn't say anything, while Olver gave her all the words of encouragement that are said at that moment. In the end, between one bite and the next, the woman dropped one of her own.

—What happens is that your mother is a bitch, I who have known her for many years before you were born, chew - I know what that woman is, only God knows what has happened in her bed. God save me from such a life.

Miss Dorothy was speechless, with her mouth open watching Olivia, who continued to eat the fruit without even making additional comments or caring what she said, Olver is standing there, looking at the young woman and not knowing how to react.

This type of action was normal, she always knew how to respond that way and managed to hit the sore spot to hurt people. Although it was strange, because on many occasions the woman was loved, shown affection or told stories, it was a kind of masochism, where some days they were affectionate and others not.

Olivia was like that since she was young, when she married Olver, she was a very beautiful woman, without wrinkles but always with that firm face, for some men it was seductive to see a woman like that, rough, she generated a strange fetish and she had many suitors, she, He would send them all away with his painful answers and they had the strange habit of becoming more attached, when he told them bad things, he would go on, asking them to tell him more things, leaving him

164

compliments and if the woman called them idiots, slimy, crawling, they would smile like idiots, slimy and crawling and go on.

Olver was one of those, but he was the only one that she liked, she was seduced by the smile, she applied the law that opposites attract. Although the woman was not loving, one day, after he said things to her, she crawled. The man said goodbye with his wide smile, but with a hint of pain in his eyes. Olivia was moved, although she didn't tell him in words, but she took his hand firmly as he left, saw his face still firm, and gave him a kiss. It would be the first gesture she had with him, because they did not have relations until after the marriage, which remained for the memory with the woman dressed entirely in white, with her veil, looking ahead, with a bad face, waiting for the ritual to end.

When he had his only son, she never gave him love, and the little one all the affection he received was from his father, who, if he filled him with kisses and affection, this balance was maintained for a long time, until adulthood. When the son knew that this was his mother and didn't care, or tried to overcome this trauma by living with his partner and trying to be loving.

The woman, never visiting her son or seeking to meet her grandchildren, was not her thing. Although she was invited many times, she did not go, even one day her daughter-in-law called and told her:

—Hello, Mom.

—Hello.

—Olaf told me he's invited you home many times, but you haven't come. You still don't know your grandson.

—I know. I know I told him no.

—Wouldn't you like to come and spend some time at home?

—I don't think so.

—Is something wrong, Mom?

—No, they're just your kids, not mine, I don't like the way you raise your kids and it's not my problem to get involved, but since I don't like it, I don't have to be there to see your spoiled child.

—I didn't know you thought that.

—There's something else. Don't call me Mom, I didn't give birth to you, not even to my son, who was born by cesarean section. You are not my daughter, you are the woman who chose my son to share her bed.

After this, he hung up.

A while later her son called her to tell her that she had overstepped her bounds, that it was a full-blown offense, and that she had to apologize. Olivia was not a woman to get angry with, she just felt the same way about what others thought, so she said no. That she wouldn't call anyone that she knew what she had said and that people accept the words they want and reject the ones they don't, if I accept what she said it's because she takes everything personally.

If son on many occasions could not stand her.

166

The only one who seemed oblivious to everything she was, was Olver, who even though the woman said things to him, he seemed not to take it personally. Although, over the years as a couple, within his own good-natured personality he knew how to give answers that the woman could not refute, then in a way they had established a habitat where they both survived without killing each other and even had their good times, because some nights Olver, in the middle of the night, would run his arm over her and put it in her stomach. The woman would not take it off, she would even hold it for him. Many times this was the code for her to turn around and make love. This ground was a place of truce where she would let her guard down and let the man touch her. Olver was the only man who had touched her and would be so until the day she died.

For any person this could be a totally hard woman, without the soul, who could only hate herself, because she breaks with all the elements of a person who deserves to be liked, she even seemed to be soulless, with an excessive ego where only what she thought mattered and what others said was worth a radish.

But this was contradicted on an occasion when her son's life began to change, for the worse or for the better, as critics will define it. The man began to have problems with his wife, problems that were so strong that they prevented him from sleeping in the house.

The only option that he had was to go to his parents' house, where they received him, he settled down and for a few days everything seemed like the atmosphere of a lifetime, the son in his room and the couple downstairs, but, by now that son was old enough and mature enough to be left on that roof. His mother had no opinion, for better or for worse, about the marriage. It was as if she didn't care if things with his wife were fixed and indeed they were.

Situations between the couple continued to be difficult for several weeks, even though the man tried to reconcile, talked to her, begged her to call him on the phone, and told her that everything had been a slip-up, the woman simply told him that this was the worst thing a man could have done to her and made it clear to him that it was all over.

No matter the pleas, no matter the plain, nothing, she was out of the house and could never see her son again.

On one occasion the young man went home, tried to enter, the woman insulted him, beat him out, and threatened to call the police if he returned. He arrived at the house with a couple of blows on him, marks from a broom handle that the woman had given him, the second blow had broken the handle in two.

Olivia said nothing, but she looked at her son, with that expressionless face of hers.

—What was so serious that you did to him? —she asked. The anger was already beginning to seem curious to her.

—Love affairs.

—Your dad cheated on me once, and here we are.

Olver lifted his head from the newspaper and looked at them, surprised by that unanesthetized revelation.

—Things are serious, difficult, Mom, you wouldn't understand.

—I guess.

A couple more days passed after this incident, when the son's wife came home, in a state of shock, without her little boy, the visit was to fight, to complain, and to get something out of the way that was stuck inside her.

As soon as she came in, she looked at Olivia.

—You, who are a mother of truth and like to point fingers at everyone.

She didn't even flinch, she looked at her in silence.

—This young man here is a faggot. Do you know why I left him? Because I found him with his so-called partner rolling around at home, in our own bed. This creep. More than unfaithful, he's a sexual deviant.

Olivia didn't say anything. She didn't get into husband and wife problems.

Olver was the only one who stood up, looked at his son with bloodshot eyes, and told him with a slow tone and a trembling voice that no one had ever felt before.

—You go right now to your room, get your things, and get out of the house. Here I will never allow a faggot, no matter how old they are.

—But Dad, it's not what you think. She's exaggerating things.

—Did you put the sausage in someone else's?

169

The woman intervened.

—No, he didn't put it in someone else's mouth, the other one's sausage was in your son's mouth.

—Get out of my house now! —I shout Olver standing up, his face red with anger.

No one said anything. The young man left in fear, his father was as never before, he didn't even look for the things he had upstairs. He went out with what he was wearing.

Olivia, who had no opinion, looked at her husband and daughter-in-law and left the room. She went out to the street, behind her son, who was walking trembling, angry, and also bathed in tears. She called him and he stopped, turning his back, not wanting to turn around, waiting for any answer from the woman who had always treated him badly, who had never been loving.

She put her hand on the man, softly, he turned and looked at her with fear, crying. Waiting for the dagger.

The woman softened his face. She looked at him and said.

—Congratulations, son, you've taken the step, and the rest will be less difficult. I respect what you are.

These were the most beautiful words her son had ever heard. They hugged each other. Olivia had a hard face, feeling pride, and a lump in her throat. She was happy that her son had come out of the closet, even if it was late.

The Cake

Chloe had been a lover of pastries for a long time, all thanks to her grandmother, who had taught her the habit of baking. This little girl, who was now only nine years old, prepared cakes, using the mixer to mix the ingredients, I would place it in the molds and ask grandma to turn on the oven, the woman would take care of the baking and after taking out the cake, when they had it on the table, they would wait for it to cool down and decorate it, they used all kinds of pastries to make the locks and at the end, they left delicious and beautiful cakes.

So the girl now made cakes by herself, even though she had insisted on making only one, which was a delicious cake and also the most beautiful one she had ever decorated. She searched the internet, checked Grandma's notes, put together a few lines, and knew how she could make the cake delicious. He also tried some of the techniques he had never tried with Grandma, but they had earrings, for future classes.

Then he got down to work, placed all the ingredients in the cup, began to beat, the machine did all the functions, and he settled down, applied the movements he saw on the Internet, which they say are tricks to make the dough even softer, added some raisins because he read that somewhere else, placed details on one side and on the other, trying to make the cake perfect.

Then, when she has everything ready, she starts to empty everything into her grandmother's favorite mold, she drains it, arranges it and waits, lets the cream be ready, and starts to make a job for her, so that when she bakes it is the way she wants it, it takes longer than recommended, but this cake has to be perfect so it doesn't matter.

Finally, she calls her mother, who turns on the oven and sets it at 333 degrees, exactly, not at 350 as some recipes say, this for another piece of advice she read, which makes the cake grow more and make it fluffier. Also in the advice is to leave it less time in the oven, to test if it is ready, open the oven and insert a knife, if this comes out clean is that it is. But this should not be done by leaving the knife clean, but between a little stained and not very clean. This way, when it cools down, it bakes to the exact point.

SHe makes all these pastes, then follows the steps with the decoration, prepares the creams, the tones and she does everything following the advice she saw in the grandmother, the empiricism, and her own intuition. She lasts longer than normal decorating, but she knows it is worth it, this cake is the most important in life, there can be no mistakes.

Finally, the cake is, just as she wants it, he arranges it, puts it in the right box and places it on the table, where no one can touch it, she runs up-stairs, goes into the bathroom, washes her hair, she has to leave it as best as possible. She settles in, brushes her hair, applies perfume, and finally, it looks just like she wants it. Beautiful. She comes down, goes to get the cake and her mother is there, standing there, looking at her with love, but also with a hint of concern.

172

—Where are you going?

—You know where I'm going.

—I want you to tell me.

—No. It seems silly to me to say where I'm going or what I'm going to do when others know, it's a waste of saliva, of time, of meaningless ideas.

—These are meaningless ideas, a conversation that has no head or tail.

—If you say so, mother. I'm going, give me money for the bus.

—You're not taking a bus alone, lady.

—Then you have to take me.

—I won't do that. You know I can't.

—But I want to go, I deserve to go, I worked hard to do this. It's my right, you can't stop me.

—Well, look at how I'm stopping you. You're not going.

—I am going.

—That remains to be seen.

The girl takes a step to pick up the cake and the woman takes it, the two of them hold the box on each side and the woman begins to struggle with the daughter and she defends herself, they push, move and finally, the woman pulls harder, the cake comes out of the little girl's hands and it also comes out of the box, it falls upside down, damaging the design that crashes against the dream and opening the cake in two, it deforms like a watermelon that crashes against a wall.

Little Chloe was left looking at her mother, with her eyes wide open and the face of a little girl who had lost a bit of her childhood in fractions of a second. She looked at her mother and began to draw a gesture of genuine hate, of a rage that came from deep inside, of a nascent hatred.

—You broke my cake!

The mother was disconcerted, out of her mind, afraid, because she had made a serious mistake, but she was in her thirties, she could not retract it, this was collateral damage, worse would be the consequences if they allowed the girl to continue with her plan.

—I hate you, Mother, I hate you.

—Don't talk to me like that," said the mother in a trembling tone.

—You wouldn't have broken the cake that I took so long to make, that cost me so much that it ruined hours of work.

—That wasn't my intention, it was an accident.

—So I hate you by accident.

The mother could not stand it any longer and slapped the little girl, she jumped up and down, touched her beaten skin and looked at her mother, with even more hate, turned around and walked to the second floor, stopped at the stairs, looked at her mother and said.

—Not even this crime that you have just committed will prevent you from doing so. You know that.

The woman did not answer anything.

—It won't be today, it won't be tomorrow, but it will happen and you can't stop it, no matter how hard you try.

That night the girl stayed awake, with one of those that prevent you from doing anything, clenching her teeth and ruminating over her mother's act, she could not believe that the woman she loved most in life had done her such a great harm as this, she did not accept it and this hurt her.

She hated her mother, that much was clear to her, she hated her very much and wanted revenge.

—I want blood," said the girl without even knowing what she was talking about.

The little girl woke up with that hate on her, the sensation of that dawn was that of sore teeth, a tense mouth.

She went down, did not brush her teeth, all in rebellion against her mother, and when she went down and her mother said good morning, the little girl looked at her and did not answer, she only looked at the table where the pieces of cake were and you could see that someone had eaten, the anger came back, stronger, she did not say anything but her eyes were the reflection of the soul. She went to the second floor again.

She would let a few days pass to put her plan into action. When her mother was neglected, when she thought that everything had been forgotten, it happened, Chloe escaped, she left on foot because she didn't have any money. It was ten kilometers away, she was embarrassed because she couldn't deliver the cake she had promised, but it didn't matter, she knew they would understand, but getting there was the big goal, so she wouldn't fail. She spent several hours on foot and when she thought that this day would be a miracle for her, her mother appeared in her car, braked right next to her, got out, walked at a fast pace, and took her by the hair that was left on the side of her ear and took her to the car and put her in it. She didn't say anything to her, and Chloe didn't tell her either, just looked straight ahead all the way, crying, a cry of rage.

For many other nights she could hardly sleep, she was going through one of the worst rages of her life, she did not understand her mother, she did not understand how she could oppose and forbid her to do so.

But she had no choice but to endure it, to accept that it was in her hands. She would have to be smarter because now her mother had locked up the house and the windows, they were locked and suffocated, but that didn't matter, because her mother was calm to have the child in, without the right to run away.

Although she managed, she was tenacious and would not let a simple lock catch her. Her mother closed everything, but forgot about the attic, probably thinking that she wouldn't go up there because she was afraid of it since she was a little girl. But Chloe faced the trauma, went upstairs with a flashlight that had a shaking beam of light, and opened the window, happy and relieved to get out of that dark attic of strange noises. She walked across the roof of the house, climbed up the trellis of plants and reached the floor, and started to run away, this time she had to take other routes, fortunately, she knew the way to the letter. She went through alleyways, crossing overstretches and looking back every chance she got, thinking about how to get there without her mother detecting her despite her efforts.

This time Chloe was luckier, she managed to get there, she was in front of the building which was her great mission, happy way, she lowered her guard, right at the entrance, behind a column was her mother. Whoever stopped her, took her by the hand, and pulled her with a little strength.

—Why won't you let me see my grandmother? —What have I done to you?

The mother looked at her, she was very sorry for her daughter but she couldn't do anything, sometimes the world hits us and we can't do anything to appease the blow on those we love.

Chloe and her grandmother had been making cakes for a long time, the girl was passionate about it and the grandmother loved her granddaughter. But as it is a law of life, grandparents end up getting sick and that happened to the lady, who fell into bed with an illness that brought others and she only had to wait for the worst.

Chloe knew about her grandmother's illness, even once she visited her and made her see-through glass, because she could not have contact with the outside, she could get sicker.

The old lady grimaced and waved goodbye, the little one did too and hoped to see grandma to give her the most beautiful cake of all, so she prepared it with all the care she could get and tried to take it away, because she hoped she had already left that isolation area so she could hug her. He missed a hug from her.

But for some weeks now her mother had been very sullen, angry, and seemed to care nothing, not even that her grandmother was sick. That's why the girl finally made it to the hospital, but was caught by her mother and scolded.

The girl would find out months later, after having insisted a lot, that her grandmother had died a couple of days after having seen her through the glass, her parents didn't tell her anything, they didn't want to hurt her, they thought she was too young to deal with death and the girl was left with the desire to share one last cake with her grandmother and playing the fool anchored with a hope that nobody had dared to extinguish.

Her grandmother's ashes had already been thrown from the tip of the Statue of Liberty. That was something she could never fully forgive her mother for, she never said goodbye to her grandmother.

Chloe never made cakes again and never ate them.

The Man Without a Face

Daphne has days having the same dream, it is not a dream that makes her feel comfortable, on the contrary, she feels that she is in front of something that repeats itself in a loop and it seems that it is not going to leave her alone.

The first night it was a man who appeared in her dreams, she knew that it was because he appeared before her and smiled at her and looked at her with that face that he loves her. The thing is that in the dream she did not see the man's face, but she knew he was looking at her with that face.

It happened in a park, in the dream, she was walking with a dog that she does not have, a brown one, she went away, approached a tree while the animal raised its paw and made the need, and there was the man, she saw him some meters away, looked at her, had his hands in his pockets and watched her, she felt a curiosity mixed with a little fear, she did not want to be stalked by a man like that.

What stood out most in the dream was that the man was faceless, everything was complete, but in the face there was a void, you could only see the other side, as if he had no head, although except for the fact that he had hair, it was straight and combed sideways, nothing else.

She could sense the expressions of the faceless man and when she knew he was smiling she was calm even though he had no face.

The man went to take a step towards her, but she woke up, the tension was great, she wanted the dream to come back, to see if she could find the person's face, but she couldn't.

That night when she slept she did not even remember the dream with the man, she had had a busy day and the dream was no longer part of her. But as soon as she fell asleep she returned again to that dream, to the moment where she was with the man, now she was in the same park, this time it is night, there is no one and she feels fear, as if she is being chased, she mixes with her boss who asks her for some papers, just as it happened in the day when she was stressed, she also dreamt about people at work, about a schoolmate when she was a child, about strange creatures and about a danger that she did not know what it was. The dream was that she was fleeing, that she was getting away from something, but in the end, she meets the man without a face, who takes her by the hand and leads her through the streets where it seems that everything will be fine. Daphne feels relief because this man found her and is helping her to reach her destination, he pushes her, leads her and when they are about to save themselves the floor opens up at their feet and they fall into an abyss, she wakes up with the feeling of falling and lasts a while awake, with insomnia attacking.

During the day she was thinking about her dream and again about this character that the first night was watching her smiling and now was saving her.

That night she did not have any dream, and the following day she woke up happy, relieved of not having to be submerged in absurd dreams. Her day's work was peaceful, she had no problems and did not confront anyone. That night, she watched a series on Netflix, and about eleven o'clock fell asleep. She dreamed, this time in a different way than all the previous ones. When he saw himself in a park, the same park as always. She felt fear and knew that she was alone, she could feel it in her chest, that it was a huge forest that it was dark and that in any corner a very big danger was hiding.

She walked, looking for a way out, but feeling that she would surely not find it. But death was everywhere, and after a while, he found a danger, the man without a face, who was looking at her from a dark space, god two steps ahead, looked at her threateningly and then started the race to catch her. Daphne started to run looking for the exit but feeling that the faceless man was very close.

Finally, he caught up with her and fell on top of her:

—Are you afraid of the dark or are you afraid that you will like what we do every night?

She woke up, agitated, drenched in sweat, had to get up and change her shirt because her back was wet and she had to sleep the rest of the night on the other side because the sheet was soaked.

The next day she had him calm, but she was a little anxious because she was worried about the way this man was stalking her, every night the same dream, it made her feel uncomfortable that she was dreaming about the same person and also that the nightmares were so strong that she woke up bathed in sweat. Something was happening to her

181

He was analyzing his life, to see if he was forgetting something, if he was overcoming some stress, maybe he didn't recognize that he was overcoming a fear, or that he was anxious about some situation in his life, that is, the unconscious doing its own thing.

But no.

That night he dreamt again of the man without a face, now he has a beige raincoat, they are in a café, it seems Paris or those who are in Italy, in the open air, in Rome watching the Colosseum. They are both sitting at a table and the man says romantic things to her, even convoluted words that she cannot understand, but that gives her much joy, she feels she is the most in love woman in the world.

When they are at their best, a man appears to sing them love songs that she does not remember either, but she likes them very much. An immense bouquet of flowers arrives, an arrangement that makes it look like a bouquet of roses. In her real life, she has never seen a similar arrangement, but in the dream world, anything goes.

He wakes up. She is not agitated, she wants to go back to sleep, because the feeling she had with the faceless man is unique, no one in real life had ever made her feel this way.

That day is somewhat difficult, and in order to overcome it, she remembers many times what has happened. That feeling of the night is what fills her with the strength to keep up with the rhythm with stoicism.

At night she dreams again of the faceless man, standing and looking at the tower of Paris, at the top, she feels at peace, a delicious peace like that of childhood when nothing worries. Later, she is surrounded by arms, which have a beige raincoat. It is the man without a face.

He puts his face on her neck and kisses it softly. They stay there, contemplating the sight and feeling themselves the happiest beings on the planet.

In a moment Daphne's mind makes her wonder what is happening, it is the strangest dream she has ever had.

The next night she dreams about him again, this time they are somewhere in the city, they kiss, it is strange, she knows she is feeling his lips, soft, warm, passionate, but she does not see his face, although she is very comfortable kissing him. She feels peace and an emotion beside this man that does not want to wake up and already in dreams she is aware that it is a dream and wants to do everything possible not to wake up.

The dreams continue to happen, and every day she becomes more conscious of it, she does not go as a spectator but decides, she walks with him. They go to a place that she chooses, as it is a dream it is as if they were teleporting, they are in a paradisiacal beach, put in a bed, hugging, kissing, undressing, they make love, she directs everything, they enjoy it and in the end, they are exhausted one on the other, while the clothes are dragged by the wind and the raincoat is hung on a rack waving like a flag.

One day, the dreams stop, they don't happen anymore and Daphne feels anxiety, every night she falls asleep with the hope of having it, but no, incoherent dreams of implausible things, she started to get angry, stressed, because she doesn't find that love of her life that she wants to have, even if it is in dreams.

Several months pass and the woman, although she still walks around with the sadness of the man's absence, already begins to accept him and at times she forgets him. One afternoon a man in a beige raincoat arrives at the company, he is the new Human Resources Manager, he is introduced to everyone and the man looks calm, with the fake smile of anyone in his position, he is thanking the employees who welcome him. He is handsome, white, with a wide smile. When his look meets Daphne's, he opens his eyes, surprised, stays looking at her, and breaks the protocol by walking to her.

To what he stands before her, he says:

—Why didn't you come back to my dreams?

They both smiled at the reunion.

My Mother

Today I have buried my mother, 73 years old when she decided to leave this world, she did it with the same temperance with which she arrived, she was born without crying, they had to give her several spankings to make her lungs start working.

She left without complaining, without saying it hurt, despite having a stage 4 cancer that had eaten away at her entire body. My mother was always hard to treat us. There was no show of love for us. Very little.

When we were babies she would talk to us in a sweet voice and fill us with kisses, but we could barely do our homework and sit down to work on our own, she started to be tough, she would give us homework and if we didn't do it she would punish us. Once I didn't wash the lunch dishes, she pushed me out into the yard and knelt me for two hours in front of a pile of corn for the chickens, and for a week my knees were on fire. I never forgot to wash the dishes again.

Another time I went out with low grades at school and he beat me up, hitting me with a strap that left me with welts on my back. I remember that it was quite a scandal, because at school they found out, and my mother arrived there, with her gallant and challenging look, at a desk was my teacher and the director, very serious, on the other side us, me sitting with my feet hanging from the chair and my mother with her feet crossed and hands crossed, waiting for the women's words, when they exposed that she had been very violent, my mother told them:

185

-I don't know how long you will live, but my children will come out straight and they will be able to be exemplary, I will raise them as they come out.

-I'll raise them however I can. The director said.

My mother sighed, thought for a few seconds, and said:

-Director, how has your son done in prison?

The woman didn't answer anything. My mother continued to attack:

-What about you, teacher? Does your son still take money from you to buy drugs, or does he already buy them with the money he earns here?

The woman didn't answer anything, she was going to comment on something, a weak defense and mom stopped her:

-I want to make something clear to you, you raised drug addicts and delinquent children, maybe because your way of love of consenting and not touching, accomplished that, I build my daughters accordingly. Let's not forget that.

That day mom slapped me, for having a big mouth, although she never hit me again to the point of leaving me with welts, I think that in spite of looking so tough, she knew she had gone too far.

When I reached adolescence I became rebellious. I dressed up as a rocker and fought with my mother, to her credit she was of the same character, so we confronted each other and her blows were only fuel to reveal more. Time passed and I got a boyfriend, I left home at 19 and I never stepped on her again.

Little by little that woman full of so much vitality was fading away, little by little after the age of fifty she had a stroke, although she still had a hard face and felt superior to everyone, little by little, as time went by she was fading away, she was becoming a soft grandmother who did not show what she was in her youth.

At that moment we got a little closer, but it would be me who would stay away because all the fights we had, the mutual humiliations were present, although I only remembered the ones she had given me, I took care of her, I was a good daughter in what I could and mom always went to bed with a full belly and clean clothes, she did not lack medicine or attention.

Little by little, Mom got sicker, finally, they told her she had cancer and this did not overshadow her more than she already was, but seemed to fill her with vigor. She faced the disease, in the first chemotherapies she would stop on her own and vomit until her guts were empty, but then she felt so weak that she had a bucket next to her that the nurse emptied every now and then.

She lost weight, she who had always been a somewhat full woman, now looked thin, almost in the bones, when she died she was just the skeleton of what she once was, a skeleton with weak skin and a nose as thin as she was.

Much later, Mom, with her cancer, advanced in stages, which was bad, until she reached stage 4 where she was only kept at peace with morphine to kill horses. She could handle this without complaining.

One day, the nurse called me and asked me to go quickly, that mom was dying, I arrived, I was the only daughter in the country, my brothers had left and they had given up on her, not even money was sent to me for all these expenses. My mother was on her bed, the one that would be the death bed, looking at me, with calm, a little sad eyes, inserted in all her wrinkles. I looked at her, and the woman extended her hand and took mine, she was cold, very cold, then I would know what they call the cold of death. The woman squeezed her hand tightly and then closed her eyes and fell asleep forever, she said nothing to me.

We buried her and I felt a strange sensation like she had lost something very big, but at the same time a relief because she was resting, with her death all the grudges were gone. Little by little I realized that mom had tried to get close to me, but she couldn't because I had a big concrete wall.

Mom was hard on us, but that woman, although with a hard word, gave me golden advice that is not found in any book, taught me about finances, about food, about discipline, responsibility, and the one I am today is thanks to her, that woman loved us like no one else, only that she was not capable of showing love with gestures, because she had a lot of pride over her, just like this one I inherited.

What I am writing is for me, but it is also for her, for my mother to whom I dedicate all my love and who I would like to give back the time to give her a big hug, to tell her that thank you for making me the woman I am, because I love her, I miss her and I need to tell her so I can feel a little peace with myself.

188

I have understood that many children feel overwhelmed by the kind of parents they have, who feel that they do not love them, but are well educated. The parents who do not love their children are those who do not know how to raise them, who fill them with low values, who neither dress nor feed them, not those who sacrifice as much as mom did for me.

I do not know what is on the other side of death, if it goes to heaven, to hell, it stays wandering and they see you as if you were a ghost, I do not know. I hope she reads these words and remembers me and makes me understand that I love her.

I haven't slept for several nights thinking how difficult it was not to say goodbye and that I will have to live with this.

I hope I can forgive myself one day.

The Separation

Gemma and Paul have been married for twenty years, both are the same age. They decided to share a house when they were 19, they were at the height of their age to study and enjoy themselves, but they had so much chemistry that they decided to live together and love each other to death.

As in all relationships, times go by and love suffers, you feel the sensations and you live, and then end up in those moments where everything is going well, but there are cracks that could be improved.

When couples understand each other's good and bad, they accept each other. They never had children, they did not go to a doctor to see who was the one with the problem and it was of the familiar situations that made them suffer, because they were left without children, then, he adopted a dog and she a cat and this way, in a certain way they palliated that ailment of not having children, they learned to see it more as a condition where both could take advantage to spend time together and to enjoy what couples with children cannot that to feel unhappy for not having other generations.

Thus, the years went by, being in their thirties already the relationship totally settled, and in the age to undertake and to look for the financial freedom, it served them to be able to make names in their respective careers and to reach economic comfort.

When they were 37 years old, the two began to have a couple of crises, they felt somewhat distant, fought for

190

everyone, and even reproached each other for what the animal had of one or the other. Just as they adopted animals at the same time, they also chose them of similar ages, so that both, old, began to have ailments. The first one to die was the cat, this plunged Gemma into a great depression, she did not sleep for many nights crying and missing her pet. The day she died she caressed her pet for a long time, felt the fur in her hand and said goodbye to it, she did it with tenderness, until she felt the cold meat of the animal and felt worse than caressing a cushion, they got rid of the body and there was no way he could encourage her, she was totally unhappy.

For some reason the woman began to feel anger for the dog, she even said that she should have died that flea before her beautiful cat, these attacks caused the couple to start fighting more and generate fissures.

The universe wanted to play a joke and the dog also died; now, it was the man who, with his soul in sorrow, buried the animal and turned against Gemma, telling her it was his fault that the animal had died because of his desires and even, to know if he had not poisoned it.

The relationship that had always enjoyed a balance was bad, far away and unbearable; he moved to another room, he did not even want to see her, she also, could spend days without meeting in the corridors and so they were for three months, until one day when the man went down for water, Gemma was in the kitchen.

—"Sit down," she ordered.

The man obeyed, looking at her challengingly, the expectation of what she might be preparing.

—"I need some time," Gemma said.

He was surprised to find himself in the same situation, he really wanted some time, he even saw it as something seductive and looked at his wife.

—I'd like some time too.

—I don't want to separate myself from you, I love you, but I propose something, let's take a year, both of us, let's do what we want and after twelve months we'll talk about what we decided.

—And the house?

—To be fair and to avoid fights let's do the following. No one will be in this house, I will go to my parents' house, you go to your brother who has wanted you to visit him for a long time, then go and occupy his space or wherever you want, you have a year off.

The idea felt good and the next day the two of them left home, canceled services, and went on the trip by themselves.

The man, happy with that carte blanche, the first thing he did was to get laid, he was young, he was in his best years of manhood and he set himself the goal of taking one hundred women to bed, no matter what they were like, tall, short, beautiful, ugly, he took them all and started collecting trophies from each one, the list was growing fast and one after the other they were a great experience for him. But after passing the 25 women, when he saw that all the vaginas were the same, that the moans were similar to each other, that the buttocks, the thighs, and even the smell were the

192

same, he began to feel an emptiness. Every time he reached orgasm he wanted to be separated from that woman as soon as possible. He was with many others but he felt a depression, the brief period between the desire for the woman, the excitement, the intercourse and ending, was a space of slight happiness, but then he was more and more sunken.

When he went to see the 43rd woman, he didn't look any further. That wasn't what he wanted, he began to think about Gemma, to miss her, he didn't do it no matter how much he wanted to, they had tried not to call each other, not to connect.

In the meantime, Gemma went off to find many things, to read, to have the bed to herself, to meet up with abandoned friends, to share with her mother, to be the single girl.

On one occasion she met a boy and thought about it, finally, she said to herself why not and went out with him, had a few sexual encounters and then sent him away, it was not what she wanted for her life, she did not feel comfortable with these worldly pleasures.

Little by little that anger she felt for her husband went away and she began to miss him. Sometimes she would see her cell phone and hope that he would call her, but she would not because they had promised not to call each other.

The months passed for both parties, she took an English course, to improve her pronunciation, he took a cooling off course and calmed his carnal desires by satisfying himself, he did not want to touch any woman, he wanted the months to pass to be with Gemma, he was even full of fear because he was afraid she might leave him, abandon him forever.

Finally, the time came, it was the day they would meet again. He was the first to arrive, he opened the door of the house, smelled has saved, went to the dining room, with the light off, they had no services, he sat down to wait, the time came where they would meet and he did not arrive, ten minutes passed and he was already beginning to be distressed, when he heard her steps, he was walking with fear, he sat down and looked at him.

Both were full of fear. She was the first to dare, she stretched out her hand, put it on the table and he took it, squeezed it, they stayed like that for a long time contemplating each other, having completely forgiven each other, he finally stood up and she imitated him, they hugged and gave each other a long kiss.

The love had been reunited, they were again the same as always, together, in love, they did not have pets, they did not have children, and it was like a second chance where it had been proven that the love had survived and that they would be together forever.

The Disease without Origin

Arlen was an incredible girl, one of those you admire for how beautiful she is, who seems to have the world in her hands and mold it in her own way. Her defect is that she had a bit of a high ego, she believed herself more than others and this had earned her the rejection of her family, who had already displaced her because she did not allow the rules to be broken at home.

For example, she dropped out of school when she was quite young, starting a promising university career. It would have been acceptable for her to have left her studies because she was going to study or do something else useful, but to go out and party or meet friends or her boyfriend on duty, no, it was unacceptable.

With this anyone can say that Arlen was disliked, an arrogant and irresponsible girl, but in the frugality of the parties the music is the only one that makes the bodies vibrate and the joy does not have to be sought.

But that is not true happiness.

Arlen liked everyone because she loved the party, because if she liked a boy she would pick him up and because in the middle of these meetings you could see her good face, the kind one, not the grumpy one that fought for nothing and that could not be contradicted.

In many occasions life knows how to put in the fold people who like to go out by the green roads and that's what she did with her, her build was thin, with light brown hair, small but round and beautiful eyes with well cared for eyebrows, her cheeks were the ones that look at the sky when they smile and her mouth was big, she hid a big smile. She was the typical American woman, white and beautiful, only she was not blonde.

Her health was good, she had never suffered from anything, except hangovers or menstrual cramps, some flu a couple of times a year and nothing else, although in her mind she was a little sick, she suffered from stress, anxiety and she said herself that she was probably bipolar, but nothing like that, she was just volatile and fought for nothing.

One day, after a night of partying, she felt discomfort in her body, she thought she had overdone it, she thought she was losing her youth, but she was barely 24 years old. In her stomach she felt a strange pressure, a stillness, there was something different, she didn't give it much importance. The next day the symptoms continued, only a little more accentuated, on the third day it was worse, she noticed that her abdomen was always flat and growing, from below the ribs to the belly, as when you are full of gas, the belly was hard and painful, she was constipated like never before in her life.

She remembered that for several days she had not gone to the bathroom, except to urinate, the days passed and she was worried, that is why she had an act of responsibility, she went to the emergency room, where they treated her, took X-rays, taken and analyzed her condition, first she was washed to empty her guts, then they kept her under observation that day and found that her digestive system was shutting down, that she wasn't doing like everyone else. They asked

196

her an infinite number of questions that she did not know how to answer, and finally they discharged her, they wanted to get out of it, it seemed that she had a strange illness and they had more patients to attend to.

Arlen had always had a habit, where she would sit, put her legs back is like putting her feet next to her butt. When she did this she felt good as if she was relieved, although she did not understand why.

Soon her abdomen grew back and she went to the doctor again, they did a wash, tests and gave her a diagnosis, they told her that her whole life had been like that only it had gotten worse, but no, Arlen went every day to the bathroom without any problem, until now.

The doctor sent her on a prescription for a purgative, which only slowed down her system further and caused her severe pain.

She knew she had to find other doctors, some more specialized than the ones who healed people quickly in an emergency room, so she began to go to specialists and they referred her to others, she soon realized she was going from doctor to doctor and finally one told her she had an illness that no consultation would cure. She was told to go to Houston, where she would be better cared for and could have more specialized tests done.

All this situation in a young woman as attractive as Arlen, caused her to be full of stress, to be hostile all the time, she felt that she could not bear to live in a situation like the one she was living in, she was there for parties, for boyfriends, to be happy, not to get punctures, medical results that contradicted each other and bad omens.

197

Every time she was in the hospital, she took a deep breath when she saw the needle in her arm coming and she was always unlucky to have nurses with bad hands that made her hurt or could not find her vein. She suffered from burning flesh when the woman had the needle in her arm and she would move it to the sides, looking for the vein.

In Houston, they checked her, did a lot of tests, and when she came to realize she was a month and a half in the hospital in a gown and connected to hoses.

Soon the first diagnosis arrived, she had dysautonomia, but that was the base disease, from there came others and it seemed that many were added. Dysautonomia is an immaturity of the autonomic nervous system, which regulates all the involuntary parts, such as the pulse, temperature, pressure, dizziness, fainting, tiredness, all this, then, when having problems. That's why she began to suffer from this condition.

But she had others, she had interventions. They put a line in her stomach, which was quite painful, to be able to empty her guts, which was the most painful thing. For a while, they used this "third navel" as she called it, in order to empty her out, but it soon stopped working.

Even though she spent a lot of time in hospitals and surrounded by doctors, they could not find the real disease, they treated her for one thing or another, and they could not find the disease.

Shortly thereafter, she was discharged, she had to learn to live with this, but she did not give up, she read a lot of content, she realized that she was suffering from an invisible disease, one of those that have no name and that doing the studies to detect it is expensive and there are not so many sick people that it is profitable. So she remains in ignorance of the medical literature.

Some time later, Arlen was already living a limited life, she had been given an electric chair to move around, because walking had become a torment for her, she went to many consultations and started to give up on traditional medicine. She realized that her disease was not something they could get in books and she had to get doctors who were open-minded. That's why they are seeing this kind of illness, but for Arlen, the economy had broken down, she had to face the conditions that her family thought all this was a new way to get attention, that she was facing everyone who wanted them to applaud her and tell her "poor girl, she's sick".

It would be several years before she could understand that she was indeed sick, her skin became extremely soft, more than a baby's, but also very sensitive, at any touch, it would turn red and burn.

She lost a lot of weight, because everything she ate she vomited and what she kept remained in her body, so, the woman who was beautiful before, now had been transformed into another type of beautiful woman, who was thin, was in a wheelchair, but her personality had been transformed and she traveled to Europe, even to Asia, with the support of many people, using social networks, talking, asking and moving to get capital.

Thus, she managed to move many other people like her, supported them, made lives where she talked with doctors, and raised awareness about the impact of the disease in a world that had no medicine for them.

That woman full of constant anger, who had an immense ego, was now simple, sweet, adorable, liked everyone, received lodging in cities where she met people for the first time, had plans to write a book, but her weakness was so great that she could not think so much, and her mind was erratic to spin ideas, but she had a clear mind to be able to organize herself and continue looking for a right to live, a real diagnosis where they would give her a life expectancy.

Currently, if she stands up for a few moments, she feels that she is decompensating and is weak, but the wheelchair has not been an impediment to go anywhere, to be in consultations since the night before. Sometimes she has to take out in a week, a Monday a thousand dollars for an exam, Wednesday 300 for another, and Friday 1900 for another, she doesn't have, but she manages to get the support and advance in a search or she keeps banging on the walls.

She, besides being a fighter who wants to get the right to health, also wants to leave her grain of sand so that one day, her name is remembered with the name of the disease, which she got the traditional medicine to find a real cure and not be a statistic in the invisible deaths.

Arlen has not died, surely she is going to die as a result of a parallel condition, maybe she will have a heart attack, respiratory arrest, cancer, gastric problems and that is what her death letter will say, not the real disease, the one that does not appear in any medical book.

Unemployed

He loved Christmas, it was the best time of the year after his birth. He enjoyed as a child to be able to buy the toys that the little ones had asked Santa Claus for, to have them at the table eating different sweets and being with the family, they always took it as an intimate festivity where they shared stories, in front of the fireplace, sometimes a snowstorm would fall and from the window, sheltered they would see the flakes that turned the street into a white ocean that would dazzle. As a child, he hadn't had the chance to share a decent Christmas, because his father was an Irish man with a weakness for drinking, his mother lived in constant depression and didn't have much encouragement to share in frivolous festivities.

All his childhood was spent watching neighbors and friends, enjoying Christmas, while he was with his pesos, with his loneliness and his miseries. Once, when he was a little boy, he went to spend Christmas at an aunt's house. She behaved with empathy, smiling all the time and her laughter made the birds that slept in a tree in the street take flight.

That Christmas at that woman's house was one of the best moments in life, the living room had decorations everywhere you looked, the lights flickered in every corner and outside the house, there was a nine-year-old doll and the whole house could be seen from space with all the lights on. That year Santa Claus remembered him because he brought him a beautiful present, a metal garbage truck that opened the doors and if you put some batteries in it when you moved it, it sounded similar to a real truck. Even the effect of the system when it chews the garbage.

That gift is also one of the best and it is still somewhere in his house. One Christmas night at his father's house, it was a TV set on with a movie on, with him playing anything, outside the house, the sound of people laughing and happy, but they, the bitter ones as they were called, were locked up and it didn't matter if it was Christmas day or August 31st or June 2nd or April 25th, the days were just as gray and dull.

That's why Rick promises himself that he will have the best Christmas ever when he's the one in charge at home. This is what he does every year, and since November he has been placing Christmas with his children, lowering the tree, opening its branches, putting up the decorations, the lights, lining the walls with all kinds of dolls, lights that sing, and even a toy Christmas tree that sings Christmas songs. Rick's house was a Christmas treat, even his aunt hadn't gotten that far, but he was happy.

The children had a tree full of presents, what they asked for and everything Santa considered appropriate to take. So there were gifts for everyone from socks and ties for him, pajamas for his wife, and all sorts of toys for the kids.

On Christmas night they played late. That night they looked at the toys, put together those that demanded it, and played until sleep overcame them. So, it is clear that for Rick, Christmas is a sacred moment, as well as a birthday, the reasons for the birthdays originated from his love for Christmas, at home, they were never celebrated.

He worked as a business consultant in a multinational company, he was already a few years and every Christmas they were always given juicy bonuses, ham, and a whole series of delicacies to enjoy at the table. That year they didn't give him anything and they were always waiting for tomorrow or the next week. That bonus was important for Rick, because with it he would go out and buy everyone's Christmas presents and what they would eat.

One afternoon a mail arrived where they announced that they would not give them anything of the delicious things they had offered him every year, it was not a bad thing to die, but then, a week later, when there were two days left for Christmas a message arrived in everyone, the chosen ones, where they talked about having had a bad year that they had to reduce many costs and among the costs were them, there he was included, he was fired without mercy, he was left without a job and there fell on him a whole amount of sorrows that he did not feel since he was a child.

He already imagined a dark Christmas, watching television and nothing delicious to eat while his children had a sad face. He did not even say goodbye to his colleagues, losing his job at Christmas was the worst thing that could happen to a person, he went out, with grief in his soul, to walk the streets and see the windows and the Christmas atmosphere, his feet were heavy while he contemplated the families inside the businesses, with bags in their hands and even with Christmas hats, the little girl with a balloon of lights, looking at it smiling, the ornament stores crowded with people, the terrible traffic, but no matter, because people were buying Christmas things and here it was all worth it, the reasons were valid.

He stood in front of a huge toy store, saw its display case and there was the train his son had asked Santa for, beautiful, from that cartoon he saw every day. He also saw the doll from the movie that had come out that year, that gift was for his little girl. Everything that was for her children was there, just a card's throw away. But he didn't dare go in for it.

He kept walking, hands in his pockets, feeling the warmth in his hands, and the rough fabric of his pants clenching his palms. He passed by that clothing store where his wife had hinted in October that she wanted a red dress that would go perfectly with that Christmas hat, saw the cake store, and remembered that he had told his children that at Christmas they would eat chocolate cake with more chocolate and see Charly and the chocolate factory.

That was over, now he would have to start the year with the sorrow of not having how to respond to his family, his loves, his wife, even to the cat that bought him the best brand food so that he could enjoy for a few days this premium food ideal for the holidays.

His mind went all the way to anxiety and he could already see himself on the street with his children with nothing to eat, even on the street because the mortgage would be auctioned off for lack of payment. The scenario was the worst of all. All thanks to the anxiety.

He walked the six kilometers that separated his work from his home, it was so much his sorrow that he forgot that he had left his car parked at the company, he would have to come back for it later.

Anyway, when he came to realize it, he was just a few blocks from his house, he saw the houses in his neighborhood and felt sorry, each one was decorated, with colors, Christmas lights, happy people inside, perfect lives that were far from the misfortune he was living now.

Finally, he arrived home, from outside he saw his two children jumping happily, next to their mother, he could hear their voices, happy, innocent of all the misfortune that was coming, his wife also looked happy. He walked to the door, stood in front of it, and introduced the key, his wife opened it, looked at him with that complicit look of support that already knew everything.

—"He called me Brooks," he said.

—What did he want?

—He was worried about you, you came out like a soul leaving the devil, you didn't say goodbye to anyone, and even when he tried to reach you in the parking lot you weren't there and didn't show up. Then he understood that you had left the car.

—Yes, I forgot.

—He called me to tell me that he feared for your life, because the most overwhelmed person was you, so much so that the others who were fired felt sorry.

Rick was very sad. His eyes burned because he could see a couple of those tears that burn.

—How is this going to happen to us on Christmas?

—Now or in any month it's a misfortune, love, but we'll get through it, we've always been able to do that.

—But we had so many plans.

—You had them, our only plan is to be with you, to be together, the children will be very happy if you give them time, they don't need more.

The woman brought him home and filled him with kisses, told him that everything would be fine and that they would get through it. That now he had to see this as a vacation for everyone. So they arranged it and Rick calmed down a bit, they spent that Christmas tight, his wife with a cooler head showed him that they had saved some money for an emergency, the fund they could use to buy the children, and with limitations to have a Christmas. That they didn't need to have a lot of luxuries to enjoy Christmas, that many have fortunes and spend terrible Christmases, and some living in brass walls at home in Latin America, lived the moments full of happiness. Christmas is not money, even if marketing sells the opposite, what is worth is family, being together, seeking happiness above all things.

The Spite

Michael met Claire when he was 17 years old. It was love at second sight, because the first time they met they didn't have a very good feeling, the truth is there was no interest between them, but once they met by chance on a bus, she came in the seat facing the window and the other seat was empty, she sat next to him, they greeted each other and started talking about nothing, about the neighborhood, the weather, and even the bus.

From that day on, he began to frequent the bus at the same time to meet her, and then he would find out that she was doing the same, taking that bus because she knew he would be waiting for her.

While they were in love, Michael felt like the happiest man in the world, he would walk to the bus stop every day listening to some happy song, the kind that fills your soul, the kind that makes you float with happiness. For example, one day he could listen to Ain't Your Mamma by Jennifer Lopez, another day a Latina by Diego Torres, so he could fill his energy and then turn it off, put away his headphones and dedicate all his time to his beloved.

They soon became formal lovers, which was to be expected because of the desire they both had for each other. Love came out of the way it is in those couples who think about each other all day long. Michael filled Claire with details, she let herself be loved and even had her spoiled moments, only to be spoiled more.

Soon, they were going to live together and the love became more intense, the bodies were in any corner of the house and they believed that it would be like that forever, but as it usually happens, the love began to cool down and they reached the stage where you test if there is real love or just passion. Michael was clear about it, he loved Claire and wanted her forever by his side, he imagined himself with children, building a future, he even had plans for entrepreneurship, because he did not want to have a miserable salary to be able to grow up, not to have economic problems, to be able to buy a house and live happily ever after.

Now, Claire was thinking completely different when the passion ran out, when there was nothing new to explore with Michael, she began to find him boring, the defects appeared, he was no longer so sweet, but a little intense, his smile was not naive, but clumsy, his voice was not slightly hoarse, but rough like sandpaper, his curly hair was not rebellious, but some mixture of a black man that remained in a past generation, and his words of love were not pure feeling, but an intense man that needed to be noticed.

Just as Claire could be loving and put a man to levitate with just the tip of her finger, she was cold, poisonous, and knew how to hurt. She managed to do this with Michael, who one day, after a silly mistake, for not washing a pot of lunch properly, claimed him, told him he was useless, that he didn't value her, and went down the path of spoilage. That day Michael begged her, apologized, and even washed the pot for a long time. But she wanted to fight, so she argued that he was wasting a lot of water that he was not responsible for, that second time it was not worth it.

208

His pleas were so much that in the end, she forgave him, but the rift remained, the fights began to become more frequent, all of them on her side, because he loved her too much to fight and to make her feel bad, but she did not care, she did not want to admit it, but she did not want him, to imagine herself outside that house gave her immense relief.

His breathing was already bothering her when she slept, his sighs, the way he looked at her, his acid breath in the mornings, having him next to her was unbearable, not to mention the moments when he was on top of her, she just wished he would finish so she could go wash, take off his caresses.

Michael was aware of what was happening, although he hoped that one day everything would pass, they would talk, everything would be fixed and they would be happy again. One day, when he woke up she was gone, only the memory rested, some clothes that he knew she didn't like, a box with the romantic gifts he had given her, and few things, hair ponytails, hooks, a pair of sunglasses with a broken stem. Nothing else. She was gone.

He took the phone and called her on her cell phone, went to the answering machine, tried for several hours, and then a message saying that the line had been deactivated, announcing that he had lost his wife.

Here began a pilgrimage where he was visiting the places she frequented, the first stop was at her parents' house, who were sincerely surprised by the breakup, gave him encouragement and told him that everything would happen, if Claire was inside, the parents were impressive actors.

A mutual friend of the two went to Betty's house, but she didn't know anything about her either. The woman was upset by her friend's behavior. He went to her work, hoping to find her, but learned that she had quit two days earlier, so he went to every place she went, including a jazz bar she went to on Fridays. Nothing, Claire had been swallowed up by the earth.

That Friday he sat at a corner table and ordered drinks all night while he watched the entrance, hoping that some of the people who entered were Claire, but none of them were. When they were going to close the place, Michael was dragged and put on the sidewalk, where he sat, drunk, unable to stand, crying like a child for his wife to name her and wonder what he had done.

Michael's life also broke down, he was plunged into an overwhelming sadness that made him feel like doing nothing, and that's what he did, he stopped going to work, when he was called in under the threat that if he didn't go they would have to replace him, he started going, but the remedy was worse than the disease, a man with dubious hygiene, with wrinkled clothes, badly worn pants and even with one shoe from each other was once, with a face full of hair, finally, his boss, who had a good concept of his employee, told him that he had a leave of absence to go for a month to recover, gave him an extraordinary vacation, all to help him, because in addition to being abandoned, unemployed.

The first week after this leave, Michael was in bed, almost all day in the fetal position, thinking about

210

Claire, sometimes trying to dial her number, seeing old photographs, not crying, it was one of those deep pains where even crying becomes useless, little by little he was sinking more into a depression that led him to the end of the abyss, he hit rock bottom. When that situation is reached, there is only one option left: to go up.

That is what he did one morning, it was not the conscious one, but his unconscious mind, which woke up from lethargy, got up, went to the bathroom, took care of his needs, and got into the shower, and the water-filled him with life. He got out of the shower and dried up, saw the mirror fogged by steam and his silhouette, passed his hand through the glass and saw the reflection, a man who did not recognize himself, went for the shaving machines, pruned his face. When he finished he looked like a different man. When he went out to the room he was surprised by what there was, disorder, the bed stained with I didn't know what, dirty dishes from many days ago, a stale smell that he had never felt in his life.

Silently he began to clean up, picking up everything, sweeping, and deep cleaning. When he finished he felt his belly creaking from hunger, he went to the refrigerator and had nothing, then he went to do the shopping, filled his cupboard and without thinking much, that night he was in the living room, watching TV, Oprah was interviewing a woman who had just released a documentary on Netflix that was the sensation of the moment, he thought he would have to watch it.

At ten o'clock that night he went to bed, he did it in peace. Right now, he was doing all this without thinking much, without planning, it was just the body automatically pulling the man out of the abyss. The weekend he climbed a mountain a few miles from home, there, he sat to contemplate the whole city. He saw that he was not far from where months ago Kobe Bryant's helicopter fell. He thought that his life was a sigh and that he was ending himself with nothing, so he came to a word that he had never thought about: attachment. At some point, he had read that this was a terrible thing that attachments make you suffer and that you could free yourself from them and be happy. Attachments to children, parents, friends, and partners, all of these served only to make us suffer.

He had become so attached to Claire that he was dependent on her, the love had withered away, as happens to millions of people every day, it was good that it hurt, but he could not immerse himself in that condition and end up with everything he had.

From that moment, he began to work on his attachments, he began to let go of things, cleaning up what was left over, to be more centered, happy, and so, later on when another couple appeared and they fell in love, he always did it without the attachment, without being anchored to a woman who might not love him tomorrow. Because love was one thing and attachment was another. He had learned this well.

Euthanasia

The day he graduated from nursing school he promised himself to be the best nurse of all, who would do whatever he could to save the lives of his patients. The desire to become a nurse was born when he was just fourteen years old. His grandmother, who was more than his mother, was ill for some years, when she was in her sixties she got a thrombosis that gradually weakened her, then she was preparing to be a senile old lady, after a couple more attacks.

For five years, she was in and out of the hospital and was everyone's burden. One night, it was Robert's turn to be her caretaker. He would stay the night, and when she asked to borrow the potty to empty her bowels. But that night she didn't, she just started making a strange guttural noise, as if she were drowning.

The woman woke him up by taking his arm and looking at him with her terrified eyes, he didn't know what to do, he moved her, crushed her chest as he had seen in the movies, but nothing worked, he was so scared that he didn't manage to call the other relatives in the house, he just shook the old woman who squeezed his arms with her hands and looked at him with her very big eyes. In the end, the woman relaxed and was left with her eyes open, and her life gone. It would take about 30 seconds for Robert's voice to come out and start calling everyone in the house, who came to see what was going on.

The grandmother was buried in tears, she was a very loved woman and the stories with her were superfluous.

213

It was then that Robert promised himself to study nursing so that never again would a patient die and when he graduated and had a job at The Cleveland Clinic, where he began working in the Emergency Department.

From the first day, he had to deal with many patients and a lot of blood and waste, as he was the new one he had to do the most unpleasant thing, cleaning up the excrements of some patients who could not control their guts. Some time later he would remember the feeling of his hands with the sticky excrements on his fingers, and going to his professional side to endure the disgust and not show the patient that he was about to vomit.

He would have to wash his hands for a long time to get that smell out. Even the gloves were not enough. Soon they saw the value he had, he was not a nurse to be cleaning up excrement and dirt, he was one who was looking for every means to save lives.

One night, a patient arrived with a bullet that had grazed a major vein in his neck, he was pale, with one foot in the graveyard. But Robert was willing to save him, so he placed his finger in the vein, plugged it and blood splashed everywhere, but he did not remove it, he managed to keep it there, he climbed on the stretcher, and was dragged to the operating room, where wet with scarlet, he was taken out while the doctors saved the man's life. If it weren't for him, that patient would have died, he was miraculously saved because he lost a lot of blood, but Robert was responsible for his not dying in the Emergency Room.

The director of the hospital found the courage that the man had, so they sent him to do some specializations so that he could go to work in the operating room, they took him out of the Emergency and he began to be where all the nurses dreamed of, in operations and in interesting cases. Now he helped the surgeons throughout the operation, he already performed some operations and even had tasks that corresponded to a general practitioner, all in the operating room, where he closed operations, cleaned and was the most experienced when a patient went into crisis and it was his turn to save his life. The doctor had not finished asking for the defibrillator when he was already holding the paddles, and sometimes he even asked the doctor to take them, because he was the one who gave the blows, this caused problems with some purist surgeons who saw a nurse as the assistant who was in charge of cleaning sweaty fronts, and handing out surgical instruments and then sterilizing whatever they used, nothing more, for some doctors the nurses were the ones who had been afraid to study medicine.

But not all doctors were like that, others asked Robert to be with them, they felt they had an important element in the operating room and knew he was reliable in emergencies.

Once, they operated on a man who had cancer, when they opened him up what they expected to be cancer in the pancreas was already a pathway of disease in the lungs, stomach, and other organs. He was in stage four and breathing a miracle. So they closed him up and took him to intensive care and then gave him the bad news. The man would be in this hospital for a long time, receiving treatments and every day being more in silhouette than he was when he entered, he lost thirty kilos and had big eyes and skin stuck to his bones.

One day, Robert came in to give him the medicines, injected some drugs into the serum and they talked for a while. Everyone knew Mr. Stuart, they knew his days were numbered and he always had some story to tell, he had been in the Vietnam War and he told how he had survived and shown bullet scars that now were a deformed outbreak on top of some bone.

The one he talked to most was Robert, he knew he had been in his operation and he said that no one knew him intimately as he did, that he knew him inside and out, literally, and told him various stories.

—Did I tell you about my Vietnamese girlfriend? —he asked.

—A few dozen times this month. —He answered with a smile.

I would laugh and tell him a similar story or tell him the same one, but with some changes.

One day Robert came to put him on medication and Mr. Stuart was quieter than usual, barely responding to the greeting, the nurse said nothing, not that it was a depression with his health conditions. As he was about to leave, he looked at him to say goodbye and the man was staring at him, waiting for him to look at him.

—All right, Mr. Stuart?

—I need you to do me a favor.

—Sure, what do you need?

216

—To kill me.

Robert's eyes opened, no one had ever said anything like that to him, sometimes in recovery he heard patients say they wanted to die, because of the pain, post-operatively, but what this man was saying looked very serious, he asked him so firmly that he felt uncomfortable not being able to say yes to him right away.

—I suppose this is something that goes against what you study in nursing school, but you are the most trustworthy person I can ask.

—I can't do that, Mr. Stuart.

—Why?

—It would be murder.

—An euthanasia, I decide, you don't do it against my will and besides I'm already dead, I just don't want to agonize, I've already suffered enough.

—I can't do that.

—If you do it, I'll leave you everything I have. I have money, houses, goods, I have no children, no wife, no lover, girlfriend or family, I am alone, I don't want the State to eat it, because it didn't give me anything after I came back from the war, you can keep it, you are young, surely a house valued in 900 thousand dollars is not bad for you.

The truth was not bad at all, but at that time Robert was looking for a house to live away from his parents, to have his own roof over his head, but the price was very high.

—I know his conditions, but I can't do it.

—Of course, you can, you just have to give a shot to that water bag you have there and that's it, something that will stop my heart, with how bad I am nobody will suspect anything and you will have your house, money and you won't have to worry anymore. Don't you mind wiping wrinkled asses like mine?

—No, if it bothered me I wouldn't have studied to be a nurse.

—But nurse or not, I know that you are not indifferent to my offer, it is a business where we win, I do not suffer anymore and you will have everything I own, without worrying anymore in life. Do you have a girlfriend?

Robert nodded.

—Better then, because you can have a roof over your head, your wife and children. What are you waiting for then to decide to do it? Say yes.

—"I have to think about it," said Robert.

—Well, I'm going to call my lawyer, I trust you, boy. We'll talk tomorrow.

Robert left with many thoughts in his head. The next day he arrived, determined, but with immense fear, he went into the medicine room, prepared several medicines for different patients and a special injection to stop Mr. Stuart's heart. His hands were shaking, he felt the metal plate where the medicines were going to be shaking, the medicines seemed to be falling, he was in a cold sweat, he was breathing heavily and he was very afraid.

When he arrived at Mr. Stuart's room, his bed was empty, he asked for him, thinking that he was having an exam, but no, he had died that morning. A fellow nurse handed him an envelope.

—This was left by the man last night. That's strange.

She opened the envelope and took out a sheet of paper that was written in shaky handwriting:

I figured you couldn't, I saved you the trouble, I still like you, I hope you enjoy what I had to build. Be happy and say no to war.

In the shadow were the papers where his name appeared and the process to be followed to make legal the possession of all the goods. He owned several properties.

Temporary Adoption

His beginnings in the world of social work come from his childhood, he had to grow up in a foster home because he had the bad luck of having drug-addicted parents, his mother used methamphetamines, and his father besides using and selling was a murderer. The last time he heard from him, he was in federal prison. When he was given a choice of career to studying, without hesitation he took Social Work, he wanted to help many children who like him suffer in so many dysfunctional homes.

He graduated with honors and eagerly began to work to attack injustice and give a better future to people in difficult situations. He helped pregnant women who had no money, who used drugs and were affecting the health of their fetuses, he helped them to have rights, to give birth with dignity, to enter rehabilitation centers, and to have opportunities for their lives. Many times he had to save the same person several times, because relapses are normal in this environment.

Many Christmas nights were spent in community centers helping to serve Christmas food to homeless people, who would spread out their plates, give them food and wrinkle their faces because they did not like the menu or those who thanked them and wished them a merry Christmas. The fact of giving a gesture to these people in bad conditions was enough to bring them a little joy.

Adam's house was simple, very minimalist, with gray walls, an old piece of furniture in the living room, an old television from before flat-screen TVs on a table full of moths. In the kitchen he didn't have a single dish to match, he served tea in a Christmas cup with a black plate or dinner on an antique plate with a Chinese landscape and soup in a Halloween one. None of that mattered to him, he had learned to value, at least he had a place to serve himself, and most importantly, a meal to serve himself.

His house had all the essentials, but an interior decorator would have had a heart attack at the sight of it. But it was his space, and he felt happy.

The same thing happened with his clothes, he wore second-hand clothes, not because he didn't have anything to buy, but because he had a lot of clothes that were given to him and he bought them at auctions, he was in favor of giving the clothes another chance. That it was bad for the planet not to rescue clothes, and he was not wrong.

One day, he arrived at a house where he was called by the emergency services, his boss had told him to go. It was Friday, at 5 pm. Upon entering the place he understood that a disaster had occurred there. In the room there was a man on the floor, with his legs and arms open, looking at the ceiling, with some cuts on his chest and a poker sticking out of his flesh. On the floor, a few meters away from him, a woman is sitting leaning against the furniture and has a knife buried in her chest at heart level. The scene was not difficult to decipher, they were used to seeing it, a couple who had killed each other. Adam's job was to go to the back room, where a child was in a corner, curled up, scared.

—"Hello," Adam said, "they told me your name is Arnold."

The young man must have been about 13 years old, very handsome, his face had some bruises, and his eyes were running away like those of a frightened animal, but also full of anger that would try to defend himself, he had his fists clenched and looked at Adam as if he were to blame for the death of his parents.

—I'm here to help you, we have to get out of here.

—I don't need any help. —The young man for the age had a thick, manly voice. He responded in a threatening tone, making it clear that he didn't want help from that stranger.

—I know you're confused right now, that you might want to be with your parents, but that's not going to happen.

—Do you want to take me to one of those homes? I don't want to go there, I know them, I went there when mom was in rehab and dad was missing, it was in that place where I... —the boy turned his voice off and put his head between his legs.

Adam knew that these places were not perfect, that everything happened here, he was aware of that, but he still wanted to help the boy. Although the system was not perfect, it was the way to go.

Adam took out his cell phone and dialed his boss, to tell him that he had to take a child at the last minute, he said no, it was Friday, the system was closed, they could not enter anyone until Monday, they looked for options, they could not leave him alone adrift, the option arose to take him to a police cell, where he would spend the weekend with other inmates and on Monday he would go into the system, but this was worse than leaving him on the street.

Finally, the idea came up:

—What if I take him to home? —he asked.

—Would you risk that? —the boss asked.

—It's not usual, but I don't see any other option.

—Nor do I.

Under normal circumstances, this would be inconceivable, but Adam was a special person in the system and it was better for a child who had just been orphaned to go to a home than to end up in jail.

—Do you want to go to my house for the weekend? — he asked the boy.

—Could I live with you?

—Just for this weekend, it is not possible to have you permanently.

—I don't want to go to one of those shelters.

—Let's go home for the weekend and see what happens on Monday, shall we?

The young man accepted, hoping to get to a home for a few days and with the hope of having a chance to live.

When he arrived home he found the scene of a patchwork set, with no definite taste, although Arnold's house was not at all elegant, the place he was in was lifeless, it was the residue of many lives, but Adam's good energy made him feel at ease.

Something he also did not have as a gift, Adam, was cooking, he always prepared something hot and ate it, instant food, supermarket food, anything. When he went into the kitchen what came out was something sticky, tasteless, or salty.

That night Arnold had to sleep on the old couch in the living room, he stayed up until the early hours of the morning watching TV without paying attention to anything they were broadcasting, just thinking about his parents, the uncertainty of his future, he was cold, in spite of the sheet Adam had given him, the furniture was hard, old and he had the synthetic leather up, he felt the stinging in his skin caused by the spikes.

In the early morning, he didn't know the time, he finally fell asleep, when he woke up the TV was off and he heard hustle and bustle in the kitchen, Adam was preparing breakfast, scrambled eggs and some toast, the black coffee was a little burnt, but breakfast was not very disastrous.

Adam noticed that the young man had a bad attitude, sullen, that he didn't want to talk to anyone, even though he tried to ingratiate himself with him, he didn't succeed. He just sat and watched television, although his mind was elsewhere, so he noticed.

Around noon Adam sat down next to Arnold.

—I just want to help you.

—I know.

—Why the hostility to me?

—You are not the first of your kind to come to help me, help is getting me into a house like that, I hate them.

—Did you suffer a lot the first time?

—It was terrible. I don't want to go there.

—If I promised to find you a good place and take your case up close so you can have a better future, would you believe me?

—I've been told that, I don't believe you.

—Would you believe me if I told you that I was once in your shoes?

—What do you mean?

—I was also a child who grew up in an orphanage. I suffered, I made suffer, I cried and I knew what the hard loneliness of these places is.

—Did your parents die?

—Mom, yes. My father, the last time I heard, was serving a 40-year sentence in a prison. He better be there, he's not a good man.

—I'm sorry.

—And I, that's why I became a social worker and I want to help you, I'm not like the others, I really want to be able to give you support, that you have a future, I'll follow your case closely and take you to a place where I know you'll be okay.

When he told him this, he extended his hand, and the young man, after thinking about it for a while, accepted it. The rest of the weekend they shared at home, Arnold gave him some cooking tips, since he had learned to cook by knocking, and they forged a kind of friendship.

On Monday, he helped him to enter a house for young people in difficult conditions and followed his stay closely, visited him many times, helped him to follow his dream which was to study guitar and to be someone in life.

When he was a famous musician in adulthood, Arnold would always be grateful to that social worker, his friend, who was like a father to him, who saved his life from the streets and from perdition.

Bribery

Fritz was the company that carried the name of his surname, was responsible for selling snacks in bags of all kinds, potatoes, bananas, sweet, salty, was one of the most solid companies in the United States and began to export the goods to Latin American countries. Chelsea was the one who was in charge of this company, she had conceived it from scratch.

It was born after her husband left her for a younger woman. She fell into a severe depression and believed that her life was over, but she was only reborn and started again as the warrior woman she is today. She had financial needs and was recommended to prepare snacks for retail, she was good at them, she had some recipes that her grandmother had left her. Her production began to please and soon she was sent to order more and the customers were increasing, to the point of having an employee to be able to cover the demand, then some more employees and at the end of a year twelve people.

This growth was bringing other types of customers, one of those was a businessman who recommended something that changed her life, to industrialize the recipe, to produce snacks, and start distributing them in stores. The beginning was a little hard, nobody knew the product, but the one who tried it repeated it and soon the brand was strong and imposed itself on many consecrated ones. Their patented recipes prevented them from copying it and thus began the real growth of Chelsea, who began to earn a lot of money and expand their plants, soon owned a warehouse and by the end of

5 years had 30 plants throughout the United States and trucks that distributed. The woman who a few years earlier was crying for a miserable man was now an enterprising woman who was respected in the country's business community. She even had a photo with Obama, another with Trump, and one with Biden.

This story could still be going well, but darkness came into Chelsea's life in the form of a man in a suit who showed up at her office, knew where she was, because he came straight to her and introduced himself as Dr. Herod.

Strange and with the alarms of distrust lit, Chelsea received the man who sat in front of her and stayed watching her without saying anything to her and with a strange smile.

—Can I help you with something, Mr... Dr. Herod?

—"Perhaps yes, perhaps no," he said in a slow voice, "I'd like to help you help me."

—"I don't understand you," she said, "I already felt that things would not go well, this man seemed to have strange intentions."

The man looked at the whole office, she had an elegant space, she had decorated it with an architect and an interior designer, she was proud of her luxurious office.

—Unbelievable that a woman who was born out of nowhere, who was abandoned by her husband by... the nanny, no... leaves a memory, by a colleague in her office, a young girl, very beautiful. Did you know that the woman left him six months after leaving the house? A pity.

All the alarms went off, she didn't expect this. She herself did not know that her husband had been abandoned by his mistress, how this man could know everything. Chelsea was scared.

—Mrs. Fritz, right now you must have all the sirens going off that say I'm a danger, but I'm not unless you want me to be. I'm just here to help you.

—Help me what?

—Help you so I don't hurt you. Well, it wouldn't be me, I don't like these things, I'm too weak to hurt people, but if a Romanian and an Iraqi who, among us, are a little bit disturbed, they like to hurt people. I wouldn't want it to come to that, surely you don't want it either.

—What do you want? —Chelsea asked, gritting her teeth in anger.

—I'm sure you can imagine, I'm an ordinary man, what our kind wants, money.

—How much do you want?

—Oh, not much. Here it is. —He handed her a piece of paper with a number on it. Chelsea took it and opened her eyes, felt her stomach churn, felt anguish, it was half of the company's assets.

—You probably think we're going to take the company away from you, but we're not. We did our math, with that money you will feel a little bit the impact in numbers, but you will not go bankrupt and you are in the constant growth of 40% per year, in two years you will be recovered and with much more money than you have now, at this moment, so to speak, that money is left over. Our aim is not to make you go bankrupt, you don't know when to knock on the door again.

—I don't know who you are, but I demand that you get out of my office right now.

Dr. Herod stood there overnight, snapped his tongue several times, and looked at an upset Chelsea, who felt a stitch in her head that was getting stronger.

—I don't want to have to tell you that my word is good and that this is something you can't help, this is something that is out of your hands, even mine, it's fate. You have to pay that amount.

Chelsea picked up the phone and dialed security, asking them to come over immediately. Dr. Herod snapped his tongue again and stood up, looked at Chelsea with pity, and said:

—I'm sorry you put us to work to show you that we are real. Because of you today an innocent person will die.

He said no more and left the office whistling. The second time security came in, she explained who he was, but no matter how hard they looked, they couldn't find the man.

That night at home, Chelsea locked the house, the windows, made sure everything was locked from the inside. She went to bed after making sure behind the curtains that there were no strange cars outside. When she fell asleep she had many strange dreams, in some, she heard distant screams, falling objects, men struggling, in others she saw herself reduced and killed.

When she woke up, distressed, and stressed by this nightmare, she felt something strange in the air. Her survival instinct made her walk slowly through each of the rooms, when she reached the stairs that led to the first floor, she found the scene, the room was shattered, in the middle of the place was the woman who worked for her, a Mexican woman who cleaned her house, dead, with a look of terror nailed to the ceiling. It looked like she had struggled. There were objects on the floor, disaster, they made a lot of noise, everything she had dreamt was real, how come she didn't wake up if she had always been a light sleeper.

The police came, lifted the body and the main suspect was her, because none of the doors were forced, nor were there any traces of break-ins. There was only Chelsea's version who claimed she was a threat, but there was the question of why she didn't call the police. Days of explanations would come, of checking the woman to see if they found signs of a struggle and Chelsea's body, to confirm the fight.

A couple of days after the tragedy, Dr. Herod appeared again in the office, this time with a smell of cheap perfume that bothered Chelsea's nose. She felt, that day she had a little heaviness in her body, she had slept badly, but the man's single visit put her on alert to see what he would say.

—Have you seen the range we have, Mrs. Fritz?

The woman nodded.

231

—The boys tell me that the woman fought, that the old woman fought. Maybe destiny was fulfilled. I'm sure you know that implicating her in the murder would have been very easy. It would be a pity if a woman who came out of nowhere, who got up after the misfortune, ended up in a prison paying for the crime of a Mexican without papers.

—Do I have to give her all the money at once?

—I like that question, I see you got the message, I have two gifts for you, if you pay us that money, first we will divert all the focus they have on you now, we will get a scapegoat and that's it. The other thing is that you don't have to pay us in full, let's get to a business, every first of the month we'll agree on a meeting in different places and you'll give me 10 million dollars, that way until you meet your quota. Better offer you won't be able to find.

—Okay.

—The first delivery will be this Friday, at an address I will indicate to you on the same Friday, ten minutes before it happens. Be on time, we don't want to show the power we have. I assure you and don't go to the police, there will be no point, we are part of the social system.

That Friday, ten minutes before the delivery, she received a call from a private number, answered and a voice intercepted gave her an address and hung up. She looked at her cell phone and found no trace of the call, it was as if no one had called her, for a second she wondered if it was not an object of her imagination.

Standing up in the place, she was cold, but with a sure face, in her arms, she had a black bag with the first ten million dollars, she was thinking about giving away her own patrimony, something that cost her to build, how much did it cost her to earn the first ten million dollars? She asked herself. One minute before the delivery, a dark blue Mercedes stopped a block away from where she was. He changed its lights, signaling to her to get closer, ignored her, turned around and started walking in the opposite direction. The car waited a few minutes and then turned on and left.

Chelsea would not give up her estate, no matter what the consequences.

The Cancer

It all started with pain, that's how all diseases begin. A silly pain that lodges in some corner of the body and does not go away with pills or rest. The pain gets worse and when it becomes unbearable you have to go to the doctor and tell him that you have a tear, medicine, and rest and then go home again.

That's what Harrison expected when he felt that strange pain in his groin, the first thing he thought was that he had an appendix problem, but he remembered that as a child they had taken it out, so he thought it was a phantom pain, some ailment of age, anything, the last thing you want to think about is that it's a disease.

When he arrived at the doctor's office, he began to check his breathing and his nodes and sent him to undress and lie down on the bed. The man, who was very professional, began to touch him, to check every part of his skin; he even took his testicles professionally, lifted them and touched them gently, touching the skin of the thighs in that area, ascending and reaching the place where the pain was, he pressed a little and Harrison released a sound of pain.

—Is this where the pain is?

He nodded.

He continued playing, despite Harrison's moans, reached a spot where a hard ball was felt under the skin, pushed it in and did not move.

The next thing was an X-ray to find a strange ball in the place and then other tests that came up with the worst diagnosis of all: cancer.

That's the worst word a person can hear. When he goes to the doctor, he expects the doctor to look at him, check his parts, find the disease, medicines and after a few days he gets better, but that word is terrible because you put a stopwatch on life, you understand the finiteness of our visit on earth.

This is how he saw it, who went home with his envelope under his arm and oblivious to everything that was happening in the street, in his mind resounded in a loop the kind words of the doctor who told him he had cancer and then as if describing the lunch menu, he told him that now it was time to do more tests and then to operate, to start a process of chemotherapies for sure.

He felt a buzzing in his head, voices, car sounds, outside noise was heard far away, only the buzzing that he had in a water bottle, moving back and forth, in his own hell. He didn't know when he got home or how long he was sitting on the couch. He already knew the doctor's words by heart and also what the papers he had given him said.

Hours later he went on the Internet to read all about his illness and came out worse than he was, terrified by that diagnosis, he found himself in his grave. He had never heard that you couldn't see anything on the Internet about tests and diseases, because they all killed.

Harrison thought about the life he had had, dedicated to working like a beast, the hard work of many hours, with

235

that he managed to build a house, have space for his children, who lacked nothing, went to the best universities and now they followed his example and had their spaces with children who also grew up healthy and strong.

But this life had only left him work and more work, finishing with the body, now, that he had barely two years of retirement, another great struggle appeared that was to face a mortal disease, alone, because his children were in another city and they were not the closest, because he had dedicated himself to work so much that he had lost them. His wife, at the time, left him, claiming that she felt depressed, that she was alone, that she never had her man, and not even on weekends could they share.

He was alone, he had never felt sorry for her, because he had always blamed the ungrateful children, who did not value their father who had worked so hard to take care of them, nor his wife who was a depressive who had gone out of the world to start her own business, she did not care at all about her husband or the family, she never lacked anything, but it was not enough

Everyone was guilty but him. But he was depressed, miserable. With cancer and he would have to face it alone.

A nurse from the hospital took him to home, set him up, and while they talked and made his bed comfortable, told him that some time ago, a patient had died of cancer and left everything to him, that now he had a child with his wife and they lived in the house that belonged to that war hero.

Harrison didn't understand much about why the man left the house to his nurse, he felt that something else was hidden there. Although he did not spend much time with him, the nurse was very kind and made a sincere effort to help him.

A week after the operation, Harrison was out for a walk and could take care of himself. When he was fully recovered, there was another ordeal coming, facing cancer, he had to be injected with the medication every few months. There, on that comfortable sofa, he would see other people sitting down, with their family members by their side, placing the medication on their arm, and giving encouragement.

Harrison was alone, at that moment he remembered his young son, who came to pick him up with a ball to play with, but he was always exhausted, with no desire to play right now. His wife would invite him to bed to watch a movie, but there was always something left to do. As the months and years went by, the children grew to the point that they simply didn't care about their father.

When they became teenagers, the relationship between father and children was damaged, they no longer shared and became almost enemies, this resentment dragged on into adulthood and now they don't even visit each other.

In these moments what he wished was to be able to meet again with his family, to give back the time and to tell them that he loves them, that he forgives them for having been absent in his presence, but that he did everything for them, he worked all his life so that they would not lack anything, but they lacked him.

During this illness, far from being filled with anger against the world, he began to feel a sadness that weighed on his back. He was profoundly weak and every night when he went to bed, he had discomfort, dizziness and after each chemotherapy, he threw up in a bucket next to his bed.

A few months later and several belt holes had been filled, he was thin, his clothes hung down around his neck, and he felt very weak all the time.

Many times, in the midst of the saddest and weakest days, he would look at the phone, hold it in his hands for a while and think about dialing a number, writing to his son, telling him what he was going through, but it was so difficult to do because he hadn't called him in many months, since before his illness was discovered, he knew that the call alone would be a nuisance, no one wanted to burden an old man with cancer, much less one who had been out of their lives for a long time.

The cancer was not getting better, on the contrary, the painful process of chemotherapies and medications that had him without hair and skin with less pigmentation were making him worse, the grades were growing and all that was left was to wait for death.

One day, he arrives at his oncologist and tells him that he will not return, that he is going home to die in peace, that when he considers it, he will call a nurse to take care of him until it is his time, even, that he knows a very kind nurse who can take care of him.

And so, months later, that young nurse goes every day to take care of him, combined with his work at the hospital. One day, Harrison tells him his story that he is very lonely, that his children have abandoned him, and that he would give anything to be reunited with them.

The nurse doesn't tell him anything, but one day, when he wakes up, Harrison finds several faces, he looks at those men for a while and recognizes that they are his children, with more weight and gray hair, men, who are by his side as if nothing had happened, giving him encouragement. The nurse was fired, but he left happily because that man would have the best nurses he could ask for.

Harrison, although he lost a lot of time of courage with his children, now he had his children loved, he asked for their forgiveness, they reconciled and the last months of the family's life helped the man to leave in peace to another world.

The Designer

In the world of design you live from everything, this is one of the most difficult professions that there is, because you have to face your own taste with that of others, when a person appears to ask for a design, he or she expects it to meet all the parameters that he or she has in mind and it is quite difficult for the result to be as the client expects, there are always changes, that if it is bigger, smaller, more blue or more red, that if it is not as he or she imagined it or as he or she said it would be.

Those who study design have this clear and when they are told, they only sigh and ask for recommendations to start over.

Donna is one of them, a designer who has had to endure everything in this business.

They have asked her to make designs with food, once they gave her an artwork of a box of chicken and told her to delete the box, because inside was the chicken, how does she explain to a customer that this is impossible, that if she deletes, behind will only see little squares, no chicken, this is the least of it, they are customers who simply do not know and when you explain, they laugh at themselves and admit their clumsiness and then ask for help.

The worst clients are those who think they know and begin to impose their design knowledge over that of real designers and have to endure a thousand changes making the work lose value and patience has to be a great virtue.

Donna once met one of these clients, the worst of all, and she had to deal with only one, the worst version of the world's clients. She had to change the design a thousand times, and the client was upset, because the art was not what he imagined, that he wanted something "beautiful".

Many of the meetings had them as a call, so the first one was:

—Hey, I'm embarrassed with you, but I have several changes that I want to make, it will be that we can make them now, are you in front of the computer? they are fast, you are an expert.

When I was telling her this, her hand was squeezing the mouse in such a way that if it had more strength it would burst. I would answer her in a very diplomatic way the reasons why they shouldn't work like that, but for the man, this was like talking to the wall because I was telling him that they should make changes.

To her bad luck, this man also took the business of making her a website, so besides the design, he took her as an SEO, who had to know how to position her, so that when people placed her name in the search engine, she would come out in the first place.

The work that Donna had to do was to educate her client, to deal with her emotions, and to come out well.

She was not a woman of patience, she had to get up many times, drink tea and contemplate the landscape from her window, she had a beautiful mountain not far away, which showed the greenness of the spring of the time, while she tasted the delicious liquid nectar she remembered all the saints of that client and she wanted with all her strength to get out of it.

When she is about to finish her cup of tea, promising herself one more chance, she reads a message that arrives on her mobile, it is the client, who complains to her about the kind of designer she is because she has just seen the sample and the text is terrible, the phrase Lorem Ipsum is repeated everywhere and she asked him to put more design into it because it is not what she wants.

Then, in the following days, after several arrangements, she talked to the client about the images, the ones that had to be worked on, and explained the intellectual property of these images. Her response was to send him one with watermarks and ask him to delete them so that he could use the design.

Normally clients have one of these defects, one, two, or at most three, but this one seemed to have appeared to show all the defects of the designers' clients together, as if the demon of the designers had appeared to make his life impossible.

They went back to the website, when Donna asked for the company logo, he told her that he did not know where he had it, but he sent her a photo of one of his business cards and told her to vector it in a moment and send it to him, so that he could work.

The nights were terrible, he kept looking up at the ceiling and was afraid to sleep because he knew he could wake up with a cell phone vibration and the man telling him to make a change.

One night, the cell phone was the one that paid for the rage, because it actually vibrated, and on the other side the message said "I don't know why you chose that font, please put Comic Sans on it".

After that, Donna's attitude changed, she couldn't stand that client anymore, she was going to throw him out, give him back some of his money and let him go and ruin someone else's life, he had already paid enough karma to have to deal with everything now, so the client, surprised by her attitude told her how could she be so ungrateful, if the design she was asking for, besides being easy, was also something she did in 5 minutes, that she even agreed to do it with her when she met someone who charged her much less, that before she had to thank for having such a good job and that would lead her to fame, because what she was doing was going to be known by everyone.

Donna couldn't stand it, she left, and she didn't answer the man. She was contemplating various options in the midst of her stress, her right hand was in pain, the problem of carpal tunnel was more intense than ever, the fingertips were asleep, and the wrist was pulsing as if it had just been hit, it was the blood running faster than normal because of the client.

What has not been told is that Donna could not dispatch the client, just like that, since she did not own her time, she worked with clients and was paid well, but it was through an agency and these were the ones who handled the clients, dispatching them, was synonymous with attacking the company and could be fired, so she had no other option but to endure it.

What went through her mind was to kill him, to make it look like an accident. She had all his details. She could arrive at his house at night, Donna was thin, her steps were light and she couldn't even feel them, so she could enter the house through a window and kill him, wearing gloves so as not to leave a trace and balaclavas so that no one would recognize her because of that purple and red hair that made her stand out wherever she was.

It was a simple job, from 9 to 17 she was in martial arts, she got to black belt in Karate, then she could be stealthy and if things got complicated she could defend herself. If the client disappeared it wouldn't be her fault, she wouldn't be fired and she could go back to sleep in peace. All of this was going through Donna's mind, because what she wanted most was to kill the client. What designer hasn't wished that for the client on duty who asks for all sorts of changes and in the end gets the first art he was taught, where the designer took liberties to help him and contradicting all the client's crazy ideas.

But she did nothing of the sort, she just took a deep breath and went back to work, making changes, modifying colors even though they went against the corporate image of the client's branding, putting the Comic Sans lettering that would make her the worst designer.

The art was slowly becoming as the client wanted it, terrible, one night he asked her to send him the editable art, so he could make changes on his own, total, it should not be very difficult to move tools and put dolls and colors. Then he asked her to make several versions. Because he wanted to see which one to keep.

Donna talked to her boss, told him about it, and told him that this was the way it was, that she had a policy of dealing with it until the job was completed. Her boss knew the client she was dealing with, she just washed her hands like Pilate and walked away, she didn't want to go into that hell.

—"Make one more change, I promise this is the last one," said the client.

It looked so appealing to sneak into his house.

—Can you put this in purple?

Walk around the house, go up to his room, wait for him to open his eyes, let the last thing he sees be his face.

—Do the design exactly like this one from a colleague of yours?

One stroke, two, three, let the soul leave the body. Go out, quietly and sleep happily.

—Can you have it for tomorrow?

Leave that house in silence, throw the gun into the sea, throw away the clothes, sneak into her bed. Have an alibi.

It was so satisfying to dream when the cell phone didn't stop vibrating, asking for changes and more changes.

Haircut

She loved to work cutting hair, she had always dedicated herself to that, as a child, out of passion she would comb the young women in her neighborhood, and then she studied to become a professional hairdresser. The best designs came out of her hands, she had a lot of demand from clients and her day was spent among lacquers, paint, and cuts.

With that job, she educated three children and took them to college, paid off the mortgage, and even helped finance the wedding of her only daughter, who married for love to a young man with few resources who had a dream of turning excrement into fuel.

Kendra's roots were humble, she came from a suburb, her father was an alcoholic, and her mother submissive, who endured everything her father imposed on her, so for her, the only escape was always the hairdresser's and the desire to one day have her own beauty salon with her name on the door. She did it, although not for free, because once, when she was starting, after buying the chairs, mirrors, and drawers to put the hairdressing supplies, she had to suffer the bitter taste of crime.

She already had a rented space, she painted it and waited for the first clients to arrive, but when there were only a few days left to open, the glass at the entrance was broken in the middle of the night and they took out all her tools. The next day as soon as she arrived just a broken wire was found, the broken glass and nothing else. All her savings went from one day to the next. Then she had to borrow to pay the rent for the place and pay it back with its fair penalty.

It took three years to get the money together to start a beauty salon again, but Kendra's psyche was always afraid of robberies, of people who are friends of strangers who might leave you on the street at any moment.

Every night when she closed, she prayed a little for God to protect her business at night, and every morning she woke up with a little anxiety, hoping that the looted business would not be found. It was her trauma, which kept her awake, that she feared at any moment that she would be left on the street.

Although her business was in a shopping center, protected all night by cameras and guards, it was quite difficult for someone to enter and steal from the business, but she was still very tough and did not allow anyone to enter and watched with skepticism those who seemed suspicious.

She, except for one time when a client asked her to pay the next day and she never came back she had not been robbed again, she took good care of it, she wanted to leave a legacy for her children when she went to the cemetery.

Destiny was born in a suburb of the city, what she had around her was violent parents who fought with each other and her mother who fought with her about things she didn't understand then, but who years later knew it was something unthinkable.

Her time at school was also chaotic, growing up in such a disunited home, her school environment made her see that she was facing hostility, it caused problems from the first day when she pushed a boy who told her something about her hair, he fell into the dirty water that came from the rain that morning. When the teacher came to complain, Destiny said that the boy had attacked her, but he defended himself by saying that he had only told her that she had very pretty hair, and indeed it was true, one of her great attributes was that she had natural, soft, reddish hair that seemed to have a life of its own, stood out and everyone had compliments on her hair.

Destiny hated being told so often that she had beautiful hair, sometimes she even messed it up on purpose, because she didn't want to be told it was beautiful, but that way, it still had its charm.

She was destined to go down the path of evil, the first acts were seen at school, when she took the pencils out of her classmate's bag, when she claimed they were gone, they began to check all the bags and to search, finally, they found them in her bag and she said they had planted it on her, but her face gave her away, they called her mother, who hid the information from her father and remained among them, under the promise that it would not happen again.

But since there was no lesson, obviously there were consequences, it happened again, she stole and this time she did it better, taking care not to be caught, she stole from the same partner and this time the tools disappeared, she threw them in the trash can of

248

another room and nobody discovered the thief and although they suspected her, there was no proof.

Her desire to steal grew as she grew up, as a teenager she dropped out of school and started stealing along with other criminals, she ended up in this gang because her boyfriend stole, so at night she would sneak out of the house and go steal stores, car logos and whatever they could get their hands on, she would do it as a fetish, and those in the gang for a few dollars to smoke joints or for fun.

The consequences didn't take long to arrive. One night, at about three o'clock in the morning, they went into a 24-hour store and her boyfriend took out a gun that she had never presented before, put it in the face of the Hindu attending the store, and asked him to hand over everything in the box. It is not known how things got out of control, but the Hindu with the dream house pulled out a shotgun and shot her boyfriend in the chest. The gun, which was later found to be unloaded, rolled on the floor and the other gang members had to lie down.

She was 16 years old when she left the correctional facility. Her mother took her to get a driver's license and started lending her, her car, rewarding her in the hope that her daughter would change, but she didn't change, she found another group and started committing bigger crimes, she was also armed, robbed and managed to make a profit, during the day she worked in a Chinese food store and when her boss got careless she took out some bills, first a few dollars, then high amounts that were noticed, she was fired.

Two nights later she showed up and stole the business. The Chinese man took out a gun that even she did not know existed, the impression was such that without thinking she pulled the trigger and the Chinese man died.

She went to jail again, this time on a felony charge.

She had to pay for three years, her face was already starting to wilt, she was living a miserable life, full of much sadness, stress, depression, anxiety and this was beginning to take its toll. She only had beautiful hair, that one had an otherworldly beauty.

She was determined to get her life back on track. She went to the mall and sat on one of the benches to watch people, to observe and think about what she could do to get ahead. She watched the businesses, in the distance a security officer watched her, her criminal face stood out. She looked at a business that caught her attention, it was a beauty salon called Kendra. What attracted her was the woman who was there, who worked on a woman's head and smiled at the mirror, chatted with her client, and seemed to denote such great peace. Happy doing what she loved.

Destiny thought that working in the hairdresser's could be a great alternative. Asking that good woman to teach her how to cut hair, to give her a chance.

Meanwhile, Kendra was cutting her hair, but she had one eye on the woman who was watching the place so carefully, looking to the side every few seconds, as if looking for the Moors on the coast, and who seemed to be giving herself encouragement to go into business. Although outside Kendra looked smiling and carefree,

250

she was anxious, sweating and nobody noticed, but her hands were shaking when she used the scissors. I wanted that woman to leave when she did.

Destiny got up, she was going to the beauty parlor, she would tell that woman her intentions, she needed a chance.

When she got up, Kendra stopped doing her homework to concentrate on the woman who was coming. She opened the door and was about to speak, but the hairdresser's alarm had already been activated and she began to scream like a madwoman, saying that a thief had just entered.

She even let go of the scissors and comb she was holding.

Destiny's fears were activated, so used to being shouted at as a thief, she gave herself away, everyone began to surround her, imagining that the young woman had just taken something, two of the salon's clients took it.

Kendra saw in Destiny's face fear, but that was not what attracted her, but all the guilt of the past, she saw in her the thieves who took her things, she saw the thieves of the world and wanted to teach her a lesson. From fear, she passed to anger, took Destiny's hand, sat her down on her chair, ordered two of her clients to hold her, and took the razor and started shaving the head of the young woman. The beautiful hair that everyone praised fell to the ground in reddish threads that died like the hair of Rapunzel, Destiny did not say anything, she cried, the hair she had hated was gone and now she loved it, in the middle of her cry she said no, please don't do that to me. But no one heard her.

When the security people arrived, Destiny looked like a military school boy, they took her and handcuffed her, the police waited downstairs, when they came out, Destiny's eyes met Kendra's, she was devastated, what she had just done. She had let herself be carried away by emotions and had ended up with beautiful hair from a young girl full of dreams and goals, she never threatened her.

Was she really coming to steal from me? That's what Kendra thought when she had calmed down.

Control

The car was considered an element that took him from one point to another, useful, but he was afraid of it, it was a strange feeling. As soon as he got in, he was enveloped by anxiety where he breathed fast and began to sweat until he soaked his shirt.

There were days when he had the desire to drive, he would get on it, start it, and enjoy going on it, accelerate, feel the engine obeying his orders and accelerate more, run. But 90% of the time he was afraid, knowing that he would be driving the next day was a nightmare, many times he questioned what was going on in his mind, he saw the variables, crashing was not fear, he even didn't care, if he crashed he would repair it, he had money, the fact that someone would cross the street and run over him was not a fear either, he knew it wouldn't happen, he was prudent.

Andrew thought about what he was afraid of, if he had an accident he would call AAA and they would come for his car and he would repair it. The fear was born of the damage that could suffer the car, that it would break down, every morning when he started it, sometimes he turned the key and did not start at the first turn of the key, he trembled, he thought he was in an accident, but he was only cold, then he started without problem, sometimes it was a problem, but nothing serious, dirty injector or minor maintenance. But the very fact that he had this condition was a reason for him to be filled with terror, to think the worst, and to be overwhelmed by uncontrollable and senseless anxiety.

He questioned himself, shouted at himself that nothing was wrong, that he had no reason to be afraid, but he was still terrified, thinking that something could happen at any time. The red light was a time to see anything strange in the car, the engine sounding different, the clutch going slower, the speed slower, going off in neutral. The car was used to move to a city where in ten minutes was going from one side to another, so you did not have to miss much to reach the destination. But even if he was in his area, he was always afraid of getting into a mess and getting into an accident or anything else, his mind full of stress imagined even braking at a traffic light, next to a truck full of logs and that these would fall off and fall on top of him. No truck was ever found and nothing like this ever happened.

His fear was such that it made him make mistakes, one Sunday, he had to go down to look for his mother-in-law 300 meters from his house and when he left the house he ran over the garbage can and ran over it, he found out when he felt something creak, he realized how afraid he was it could be dangerous, if it had been a dog, he would have killed it, if it had been a child, he would have been in prison for involuntary murder.

When he had to go out to the other city, which was two hours away from his own, he was filled with terror, it was taking the highway, in his mind, he had to cross a few miles without coverage, that this highway was supposed to be dangerous, that sometimes the injured were robbed, that he could lose control and go through one of the gaps on the sides and fall down and explode like the cars in the movies.

The curious thing is that the fear began when he knew he had to use the car, he began to suffer and see the time, knowing that at a certain time he would have to get out in the car, but just when he got in, he felt high anxiety, dizziness, sometimes he spat out, he sweated in spurts even when he was just bathed, he turned the key and when the car started it was as if the purr came from his mother's womb telling him to calm down, then the anxiety would stay, but with less intensity than before.

Sometimes when he was driving for a few hours in the car, he didn't want to come back, he wanted to keep driving and he would go on the longest routes to enjoy himself.

Another trauma that he always had was the fear of running out of fuel, it was dread, that the tank would empty in the middle of nowhere and he could not help himself. No one likes to be in an accident, but Andrew's terror was similar to that of going to the scaffold. Every time he went out before returning home, he would fill up the car, put gas in it, sometimes passing by the station early, and when he returned, the same man would attend to him, look at him strangely, and put in a liter or two of gas, he hadn't spent any.

Already this evil could be considered terrible enough to have no aggravating factors, but soon he began to suffer more, when he was going 50 miles per hour he felt that he could crash at any moment, or the car for mechanical reasons could be divided in two and be at the mercy of physics and crash into a wall or run over other people.

On other occasions he was afraid of losing control and dying or running out of brakes, under normal circumstances what would be expected of him is to brake, to go less than 50 miles per hour, but while his brain was telling him there was danger and cortisol was flooding the body, his foot accelerated more and went over 120 miles and more, while the fear was increasing, all the way to a stop at a traffic light, which gave way to an anxiety looking for the strange sound of the engine, all normal, he breathed a sigh of relief. The tension was in the cusp, he pressed the steering wheel with such force that for the rest of the day his hands hurt from the force he was exerting.

Many times he smelled his hands, looking for some strange smell that was coming out of the car, maybe burnt oil, overheated engine or so many things he had read on the internet and could have come from a broken car.

Just as on the internet or you can read about health because everything is cancer and it is terminal, you cannot see a symptom of the car, everything is expensive, deep damage and that can be the whole life of the car in danger when it is nothing more than a loose nut or an imbalance in a tire.

But Edward looked at the internet and was filled with fears and started tying up loose ends, giving a reason to the post he read, saying that in effect the car was about to burn, that when he least thought about it he would light it up and black smoke would come out, or in the middle of the highway fire would come out of the hood and he would be left looking at the metal torch.

The material didn't weigh him down, if he burned himself it was even a relief, he would get out of that car, which wasn't bad, it just failed in his mind. The mechanic would look at it from time to time and receive money almost free, because what he did was dust it off and look at the oil, everything was always in order, with few exceptions and they were damages that any car owner could fix, anyone, except Edward who considered that metal box with wheels an enemy that had come into his life to mortify him.

He would sometimes pass by the garage and give life to the car, look at it off and imagine that it was looking at him, waiting to kill him, like the cars in that old Stephen King movie, inspired by one of his books, but in this case it was not going to kill him by running over him, I wish death was that simple, this car was more cruel, it would get into the cracks of your mind, looking for its deepest fears to get them out and torture it to the point of reducing it to a man's pinky, to a piece that was useless, that would be terrified as in hell itself, being submerged inside it, using it, leaving it with loose ideas that it could be damaged or something could happen to it, what? I didn't know, but anything could happen.

Edward's fear was one of the strangest of all because he was not afraid to drive, he considered himself good, he even had reflexes that came out of his own anxiety, so he avoided a crash where in other circumstances it would have happened.

The car was always in optimum condition, with him I would have been able to drive across the United States from one end to the other, the tires were perfect, I could see them every week, his air pressure was

257

correct, it was aligned, the engine oil was new, he changed it long before it was necessary, the engine purred again, everything worked perfectly, but his fear was immense and he could not afford to enjoy the car.

His fear was born from other inner fears, from insecurities, but he did not know it, he considered himself superior in many things, remarkable, he was only afraid of a car that had never given him any reason, of something new to him.

He would continue to excuse himself that it was the car, that when he bought the agency car he would leave behind his fear, his insecurities, but when he was able to do so, years later, he suffered the same because he feared that he had been swindled, that the car would come from the assembly company badly, that the one-in-a-million engine would fail, that the tires would wear out asymmetrically.

His fears were great, they were terrible and they would accompany him all the time while he was behind the wheel, because not even his psychologist was able to heal him, he only gave him some relaxation exercises that he tried while he was driving, they were of some use, but his body was sweating, his breathing was agitated and his knuckles were white from the strength of the steering wheel.

Some fears are in the DNA and cannot be removed.

The Photo

The family got into the car, three people were on board, of those three, only one person would return, the others would never be seen again. Austin knew this, he recognized that he was leaving forever, but he didn't want to think about it. He saw the cab leave and one of the crew members turn around and wave goodbye, the other two didn't even see him. He entered the house and stayed with that immensity all alone for him and two cats that were not even his own.

They had not even left the neighborhood and he found the house so big, so empty, and full of so many memories painful. He went up the first stairs that separated him from the main door, to his right there were some stairs that led to the other floor, where two of the inhabitants of that house occupied, those who would never return, inside, the other person and he lived.

He entered and saw the fish tank, three sad fish were spinning endlessly and all you could hear was the motor that gave oxygen to the aquarium. He walked down a small corridor until he reached the kitchen and at the top, a little more than two meters away, was an old parrot, which he could not see out of one eye, but had been his companion in that house for more than two decades.

He walked around the house, reached the back, where there was once a working life and now there was only loneliness, stopped machines, poverty. Everything had been extinguished in his life over the years. He went down slowly, walking without much plan, he arrived again at the living room and contemplated the stairs that lead to that annexed floor, he thought about it for a while and dared to go up, when he arrived upstairs he found a bed that was recently occupied by one of his relatives.

Now empty, it was only a stained mattress of so much use, a bathroom without water, a broken light bulb and a second-hand baby cradle that would never be used by that little boy, his grandson would never sleep in that room again, nor his daughter. He saw a white paper painting next to the bed, he walked over there, hoping to find some valuable information, to call his daughter, to tell her to come back, that there was some valuable information, to ask her forgiveness, so she wouldn't leave forever.

He picked up the paper, it was a picture taken from an instant camera, in it was him, Austin, with a baby in his arms, his grandson, he was laughing, the picture had been taken by his wife, in fraganti, in the collection of his daughter's things, that picture had been less important than anything, it was thrown away like garbage.

When had it all gone to shit, thought Austin, when had he lost his family?

When he was young, he wanted to have a family and do things differently. He was born a bastard, his mother had had the audacity to roll around with a man from the countryside, she had gotten pregnant and he came out of it, the other brothers were white, blue-eyed and their skin wasn't dark, but he didn't have their light pigmentation either, his mother had slept with a Mexican, the result was a dark-eyed brown with his mother's hair. A combination that never pleased his siblings, was always the displaced one, the lover's son.

When he grew up he left the city, moved to Texas, where he started working on whatever came his way and finally set up his business, a big grocery store that he managed with steel tempering for years, they produced many things in the back of the house and in this place there was a dense, heavy air that suffocated and everything was a product of him. His daughter had to be there, who suffered mistreatment, words of contempt, and even beatings. There was never any affection that treated her well and she felt that she had an enemy instead of a father.

Soon this manifested itself in her personality, she started going out with several boys, looking for paternal affection in whom she was nothing, fell in the arms of furtive lovers, in the arms of married men, and gave herself to pleasures of every kind that after compliments left her with a void in her soul. Finally, one of those many men brought her a pregnancy that had given birth to that baby, her father during the whole pregnancy judged her, called her a whore and other offenses more, she, endured in silence all these blows, waiting for her moment, tied hands.

Finally her luck had come, a chance to work in another city. From one day to another he organized the trip and left when he got into the cab the only one who said goodbye was his wife and baby, his daughter did not even look at him, as if she did not care, this broke his heart, hurt him deeply. But he said nothing, his pride allowed nothing. He left.

There Austin was now, lying on the floor, with the photo in his hand, remembering the baby, the day of that photo, wanting to be able to live those moments. Sometimes mistakes are made that cannot be corrected.

Already Austin was an old man, he was at home, depressed, knowing that for this life he would not be able to see his daughter, nor his granddaughter, he took the phone and wished he could tell the young woman that he loved her, that he forgave her, but no, he began to weave reasons, to say that she was the guilty one for not being a right-winged young woman, straight as he was, but he forgot that in his youth he had a son with a woman and abandoned him in that city and he never heard from him again. Nor does he remember that he was not the most responsible, that he had an age where mistakes were made, but nothing, he only remembers how upright he was and that no one guided him.

Although now, immersed in this sadness, he only thinks about the fact that he lost a great opportunity in life, his daughter enjoyed it the first years, when they went out to walk, play and walk, then when she grew up, the relationship became more distant as he tightened the screws and became more radical, strong and violent, the girl was afraid of him for a long time, she was afraid that he would give her many blows, it was that crushing power that gave her terror, but later the fear also gave way to rage, the two were added together and in the end, the last one prevailed and the way to challenge

262

him was by doing what he did, breaking the rules and creating a harder war.

What is the use of having a war with your children if in the end you will end up alone, with your children far away?

Austin crumpled the photograph up tightly, with hate, felt the texture of the paper ball in the palm of his hand, carved it. He opened his hand and put the photograph back, and filled it with kisses, apologized while crying.

He knew they were facing a difficult situation, where they had to face that departure as soon as possible, so he told his wife to accompany her to Cleveland, where his daughter will now live, and to spend Christmas there, also in the New Year. For the first time in more than thirty years, he will spend the holidays alone, with a house so neglected that it falls apart, with leaks, humidity, and damage everywhere you look.

On Christmas Eve, he sits on the balcony of the house and looks at the city, all the houses are lit up, with families laughing out loud as they share dinner and drink, and his house is dark, in silence. He ate the cereal in the morning and some mashed potatoes with a little sauce at noon. It does not provoke him to eat, he just wants to die, he no longer has any reason to remain in this situation of depression and loneliness, why, he lived for his daughter, he worked so that she would have a future, and now he has only the hope of a short life where he will end the suffering.

Meanwhile, his daughter and the little one are settling down in the new city, her mother is helping her to adjust to her new job and is taking care of the baby in the meantime. Time passes after Christmas when the woman returns home. She wants to meet her husband again, she misses him, she has time without seeing him, and when she arrives all she wants is to see him so she can share with her husband.

When she enters, everything is silent, she calls him, waiting for an answer. She does not get it, walks through the house and does not find him, finally goes up to that annex, where her daughter lived, and when she arrives upstairs she finds him, he is on the ground, lying on his side, has in his hands the photograph, his eyes are open, she comes closer, touches his foot and it is frozen, his soul has gone for a long time, he has died, he has not endured living with so much pride and preferred to die rather than give in and fix things with that part of him, the daughter.

He chose the exit of the cowards, his daughter would say soon after, but her mother stopped her and told him that if he had been proud, she would not stay behind. Regardless of who the culprit was, in that tomb rested a man who suffered from deep pain and died of love.

Sometimes pride is stupid.

The Accident

She had an electric car, one of those that you don't know if they're running or not. She loved speed, put her foot on the gas, and loved to mute, without listening to herself, but at 150 kilometers per hour on a highway. The best way to drain was to drive her car, she loved it, she did not suffer from fears.

She had worked all her life as an accountant in a company, she had already retired and now she was at home, enjoying her last years. She would go out in the car to get the groceries, to bring the sand to the cat or its food, or to go to the park a few miles away to walk the dog, she was a body full of energy not to stay at home, like an old lady, making cakes and knitting socks.

She had been a widow for five years, now, with the house all to herself, she missed her husband, when he died of a heart attack she was given a leave of absence, but she did not take it, she went to work, and there she gave herself up until the day she retired. Then, when she was home, she started looking for what to do with her life, the first thing she did was to find entertainment walking the dog, doing crafts, and driving.

Soon after, she received a call from her only son, who told her that she had to travel to the other side of the country to fulfill a mother's duty that she could not refuse. She tells him so, that it is a proposal she cannot refuse because she has to be present at his wedding with his lifelong girlfriend.

265

This was one of the happiest moments for Indiana, who prepared everything to go on the trip, organized the suitcases, the dresses, the shoes, went shopping and in two days had the car full of all the things he would take to the capital. She started the trip one day at 6 in the morning, she climbed into her car, put on Phil Collins' playlist, In the air tonight, the song started softly, while she put on her dark glasses on her head, waiting to put them on in a while when the sun attacked, she set out on the road, this time she wouldn't use the electric car because then they weren't so developed to enable them for a long trip, she got into her husband's old car, a Mustang, she was excited, she loved the noise of the car, the roar. As soon as she turned the key she jumped up, faithful as any Mustang this one turned on, she had already taken it to the mechanic to confirm that it was in order.

She went out to the highway, listening to Phil Collins still in his long, soft intro, thinking that she must have put AC/DC to ride in this car. But Collins delivers, the battery rings, her foot tickles, she pushes the Mustang a little harder, and it responds by moving a long way in seconds. When she took the highway she was going 140 kilometers per hour, with a car that went from 0 to 100 kilometers in just three seconds, although she still had trouble mastering it a little, because this was big compared to her electric car that was smaller than a Volkswagen Beetle, after noon she was singing Metallica songs that she put on the cassette of her husband's old radio.

The long highways of America can be boring, endless flat roads without a soul along the way, have been the inspiration for countless horror movies. The only thing

266

left to do was to run, and that was what she was doing, having her foot almost at the bottom, feeling the engine moving without a single complaint because of her demands, setting as her goal to reach before the arms of her son and her new daughter-in-law.

She imagined the wedding, the church full of balloons and flowers, the tall son in his formal suit and the bride in her beautiful long tail dress, with all the relatives filling the pews of the church, with a joyful reception, hoping that her son would grant her the opportunity to dance a piece with her, to give her his blessing of her new life.

She stopped at a restaurant on the way, had lunch, received compliments from a trucker's car, and continued the journey, a couple of hours later it happened. Despite having several hours onboard that car and driving it well, she had not noticed that one of the tires had a problem, the rear left side, was going at a speed of 100 miles per hour, singing the song of Tarzan that Phil Collins composed many years ago, the wheel fell off. It passed by her side, the steering wheel suddenly went crazy, she tried to control it, her instinct made her put her foot on the brake, she sank it to the bottom and the car crashed, she went around one turn, a second turn, three more, she stopped on her head and fell on her roof, in the middle of nowhere, occupying both channels. It was totally destroyed. Surely the wheel had loosened up and she fell, at that speed and the bad reaction she was now unconscious, bleeding and with a car about to catch fire.

A few minutes before she had passed a van carrying vegetables, this one when reaching her saw the result a man with a straw hat and panties got off, ran and helped her out of the car, placed her on the side of the road and called Emergency.

The wedding paused for a few months, while she recovered, a broken arm, a leg, bruises, a hard blow to the head. She had come out fine for the intensity of the accident, otherwise, she would have died of burns.

The memory of a mother with one arm in a cast, with her face still a little marked, but happy, would remain forever. Indiana spent a few months at her son's house, just getting back on his feet. When she felt that she was the mother-in-law who was invading the intimacy of some newlyweds, she decided to leave, she went to rent a car to return home, she was doing well, comfortable in search of the car, but when she got on, she was left with ice, looking at the steering wheel, with the key in her hand, she felt a sensation that she had never had in her whole life, a paralyzing fear. Her hands could not hold on to the wheel. She had to get off and run to the entrance, where she emptied her guts, she couldn't travel by car, she decided to take a plane home.

Here she would begin a procession to learn how to overcome her fear of the car, she did it with her electric car, with which she felt confident, she would get in, start shaking with fear and get out again, every day a little. Indiana was not a woman of getting her hands tied, bearing the crises, she took them by the neck and began to solve them, this stress and fear caused by the car began to overcome it little by little. She would try to spend as much time as possible in the car, she would get in the car with her cell phone, she would put on some Netflix and she would enjoy it for a while, then, already relaxed she would eat something, it was very difficult for her to get to that point, she would decide to get in, she would procrastinate all day long getting in the car, this was suffered by her pets that now did not go to the park as before.

When she overcame her fear of being inside the car, she began the process of getting in, staying there, taking breaths of relaxation as she had seen on the internet, then she would put the key in, or try to because she was shaking so much that it was difficult to get in.

On the fourth day, she did it, she stayed there, breathing hard, thinking about whether to turn it over or not. One day she turned it, nothing happened, she realized that the car had been unloaded for weeks, she smiled willingly at herself, a loud laugh that only amused her.

The next day, certain that the car was loaded, she got in, repeated the ritual of turning it back on, turned the key and a soft buzz announced that she was ready to go. She gently touched the accelerator and the car moved a few inches, turned it off, and stood for a while breathing, controlling the urge to vomit.

Little by little she got out of that fear, the first days she began to drive slowly through her own neighborhood, sometimes laughing at herself, because the one who some time ago was sinking the accelerator to the bottom, with one hand on the window, like those men of the last century in convertibles, now was a little old lady who had her hand in the position of the hands of

269

the clock, in 10 and 2 and was driving at 40 kilometers per hour.

Soon she dared to go to the supermarket, arrived, did the shopping, chose her own provisions, and did not depend on the household that brought her tomatoes as she did not want them or the abused fruit, she had everything just as she wished. Although while she was doing the shopping she thought she should go home, she would have to drive again.

The first day was the most difficult, she soon returned to her routine, taking the dog to the park, doing the shopping and driving, she stopped doing it at a slow speed, she did it a little faster.

One day, coming back from shopping, she entered the highway, felt the itch of her foot, and dared to accelerate, ran, and felt the adrenaline.

Fear of Death

We all have fears, of heights, dogs, cats, spiders, closed places, and even of water, they disguise them as phobias. There is one that is collective, the fear of death, we all fear death and that is why we have the instinct of survival, if we fall we put our hand in, if we go back we put our head forward to protect our brain, it is part of the instinct and practically all animals have this instinct.

Although there are some fears of death that go beyond rationality and nature. That was the fear that the protagonist of this story had, who protected himself above all things from dying.

His terror began when he was eight years old, when he was riding a barbecue on a bicycle and accidentally got loose from his uncle who was riding at full speed, he fell and hit himself a lot, he was unconscious for ten minutes, when he woke up he had wounds everywhere, he had lost several teeth, and he was left with scars for life. The doctor told him that it was not his day that he could have died.

Hopefully, he healed and had no aftermath except for scars on his body. But in his mind he was left with a very strong fear, that of dying, he began to take care of himself with a fanaticism that as he grew up made him stronger.

As a child, his habits were never to ride a motorcycle again, and even on a bicycle, he would become an old man without being able to climb on a bicycle. When he was on the school bus, he could not see the movement through the window, so he would sit on the seats in the aisle, and he would see the floor of the bus or a classmate, never through the window, missing the landscape of the road.

Later in his adolescence, he would not cross a street until he saw other people going by his side, helping him cross. But if a traffic light was red with all the cars stopped and he was there, he would stay there, looking at the drivers who looked at him as if he was an idiot, losing his light to cross.

Every night when he went to bed and was about to close his eyes he thought that if he closed them tomorrow he might not wake up, he would fall into a possible abyss that would plunge him into eternal death. The next morning, when he opened his eyes, he was happy to be alive. He took the time of sleep as a way to death and did not control anything of what happened. So what was around the bed he removed, he was afraid that if by bad luck there was a tremor, the ball he had on a shelf would move and fall on his head or temple and kill him, or the tennis trophy would fall on its edge, bury itself in his eye and kill him, even though he had all these cares, he could not ignore that he could die if there was a natural tragedy, an earthquake, and a wall fell on him. So every night was an adventure for him, a game of adrenaline, a thought of whether or not he would wake up the next day.

There were nights where he woke up scared, looked at the darkness, and stayed trying to decipher the shadows, thinking if one of those could appear before him and kill him, he stayed with those fears until he fell asleep.

When he reached adulthood his fear was accentuated, everything began with a health class at the university, where they told him about dangerous foods, the first on the list were the processed foods, he immediately abandoned all processed foods and also some healthy foods that he investigated could be murderous, for example, he did not eat more apples because he feared that he could eat the seeds that had cyanide and die, although he read that he would have to eat the seeds of 18 apples to be dangerous, anyway, he abandoned the apples forever.

He did not consume any sugar and salt, just the seawater, he began to buy sea water to prepare all his food, because he had read that this way he could prevent many diseases, so his house had bottles of seawater to prepare the food.

This had its benefits because he began to enjoy the flavors better, thanks to this technique, although this could be good, he did go to the extreme with other foods, he stopped drinking natural fruit juices because he read that these had a lot of sugar, he only consumed one piece of fruit of each and maximum three a day, he ate many vegetables just boiled.

He stopped eating processed cereals, and all his food became that of a monk; this left him as a result a healthy body full of vitality, as for energy, he processed it with sport, but always with exercises that did not represent a risk for his health and always controlling his heartbeat; he did not want that by an excess he ended up dead of a heart attack.

All of this would have been fine if the fear had not been accentuated to other fields, such as anxiety, although he had all the care that a person can have, he did not have relations if it was not with a double condom and some women even asked him for an STD test, he brushed several times a day because they told him that a cavity could cause a heart attack. He took care of everything, he was the safest man in the world, but he still had anxiety, he suffered from anxiety that was combined with control exercises, slow breathing, trying to calm down, but this was like taking water out of a leaky canoe with a bucket, he never finished.

He always had obsessive thoughts about death, had taken the habit of seeing things and imagining how it would be to die there; for instance, if he found a piece of pipe coming out of the ground, he imagined that by accident he stumbled and fell on it, buried it and died, If it started raining he imagined that his feet slipped and he fell hitting himself on the back of his head if he saw a fire, he was afraid that for some reason it would fall on him and he would be totally burned, if he was in a car he imagined that he was hit and would be thrown out of the glass and die, so when the duct accelerated a little, he would brake with an imaginary pedal, he would become anxious.

All this also had an aggregate, frequent depressive pictures, he would sink in a deep sadness, where he believed that he would die of sadness at any moment; he used to stay in bed for several days, curled up, in a fetal position, and feeling that coming out of that padded rectangle was to get into danger. The anguish did not allow him to live in tranquility.

Sometimes, when it was unavoidable, he had to expose himself to some danger, he had to cross a street, eat some processed food because where he was he could not avoid it, he had to drink cold water that did not do it because somewhere they had told him it was exposure, that it froze his fat and could give him a disease that would kill him.

Anything as insignificant as it was, if he considered it a danger, it would plunge him into a terror that would make him suffer panic attacks that he could not control with anything, people would try to calm him down, but he would scream more and become an upset person who could not control himself. Sometimes they had to calm him down with water and hug him, tell him everything was okay and help him breathe, but this was so frequent that his family could barely stand it.

This paranoid life had prevented him from having partners, friends, a girlfriend, anything, he was alone, except his family.

One day, his distraught mother asked him, for God's sake, to seek help, to go to therapy, if not, to put his hand on his heart and understand that he was doing something crazy, that it was not normal to be acting that way.

He began to read books about curing fears, and reached the fear of death, he documented this and gave himself more to meditation and yoga, this was helping him little by little, added to cognitive behavioral therapy that made him go healing little by little, it touched him many times to face the fear of death, see it closely along with all the fears that it brought, only with the purpose of overcoming the fear.

Years later, when he already seemed to have overcome it, his mother died, a natural death, he was of advanced age, it happened as a joke of the universe, while he was at home, he had to see the body of his mother there, in his bed, resting as if he was sleeping, standing before the body, the man trembles, people who are afraid of death cannot see dead people because they become unbalanced, they feel that they can lose the sense of control, this is what happened to our protagonist, who was standing before the body of his mother and all the fears returned.

The woman or the body that she used on the earth began to have a reaction, she opened one eye slightly, the product of her process of decomposition, but the glass of the eye seemed to look at him, this took it as a sign from her, that she was asking him for strength to go on and also order, to leave as soon as possible from there.

To the annoyance of his family, he did not attend the funeral, went home, hugged his wife who was understanding, and cried for a long time, then she, on his behalf went to the funeral.

There are fears that are difficult to overcome, that hurt and although they are controlled, they remain present and are likely to surface at any moment. That day when his wife was at his mother's funeral, he preferred to throw away his favorite, processed yogurt and took a piece of watermelon, the best thing was natural, unprocessed food. He took all the seeds out of the fruit and ate it. As he remembered his mother.

The Bottle Draining in the Sewer

Hello, my name is Barden, I'm an alcoholic... in the mind of each of you must have sounded the "Hello Barden" said by many voices as if it were a double-A date. I'm an alcoholic, but I didn't know it, for years I was falling into an abyss until one day I realized that this was real and I was sunk to the bottom. I had to emerge and slowly learn to accept myself with my faults and virtues and of course, put the bottle aside.

Although let me tell you that I drink, but I am not an alcoholic, maybe now you see me with skepticism, I haven't been drunk for years and I don't have the desire to drink either, only if you invite me to your house, serve me a beer, two, three, ten, we drink them, I will get a little happy, I will go home with a little hangover and that's it. It wasn't like that before, I went through a hard time in my life and I want to tell you about it right now.

This world is strong because when you're inside you don't even know it, when you come out you realize you've made a series of serious mistakes and you're in trouble. You do all of this to be able to cover up deficiencies, to pretend that you have done bad things. The truth is that now that I see myself, at that time my self-esteem was not the best, I felt insecure about many things and some people do not know it, but I lived with fears, with anger and I hid it with a smile, but more than once I crashed my hand against some mirror and I saw my blood, I had a desire to hit, and this calmed it with liquor.

I had two stages with the liquor, one was where I drank and had fun, when I started drinking I felt extremely comfortable, then, life became more bitter and I drank out of bitterness, that's where everything starts to get complicated in my life. At one stage you feel the most fun, at another, you feel shitty.

Without any problem I could drink 15 liters of beer a day because that was what I liked most, beer, then I could drink everything, I even drank like water one of rum, and if I could not more, I ran to the bathroom, fingers to the mouth and continued drinking. At some point I drank everything like a thirsty drink of water, from the spout of the bottle, I was the typical bearded man with a bottle in a paper bag.

It wasn't that I started drinking and fell into alcoholism, it was a gradual process, I think it took me years to end up an alcoholic, I started as a child, I was in school when I was just twelve. It was at that moment when I tasted the first drop, I lived in a bad environment and the only thing I wanted was to drink and be happy for a while.

At that time I drank when I met friends, when we had parties, it would be my father who would give me the first beer, I was fourteen years old, she was the celebration because I had just opened as a man with a kind prostitute who took me to her room and made me everything. I started drinking with my father without knowing that it would lead me to end up in an addiction.

I suffered for a few years from being overweight, I was the fat one in class, they picked on me, but when we drank I wasn't the fat one, I was just another one, I was something with a big mouth that sometimes ended up getting beaten up. But then we would make up, liquor has that gift of bringing friends together and separating them while they drink.

The only constant thing is change and the school moments are over, those people who were with me in school ended up badly, of the ten of us who were in the group, there are only two alive, one is me and the other is one who managed to transcend and today is a senator. We never talk again.

Dad was an alcoholic, I know, at the time I took him as a nice man, nice who laughed a lot and gave me one beer after another. My father died of cirrhosis, so would his passion for liquor. As for me, at home there were many rules, they let me do what I wanted, but they controlled my food, they made me go hungry, as if that would solve the fatness that was. I would sneak out at dawn to eat cookies and milk in the morning, so I always got fatter and fatter, despite their controls. Anxiety was treated with food, another one of my addictions.

All this led to my 23 years old having to go through surgery to lose weight, I was almost 200 kilos in my 1.80 m height. That was my time of healing, I didn't take a drop, but one Christmas I was given a drink, and this one was linked with another and another until I ended up totally drunk.

As a young man, I drank and had a good time, at twenty I bought a house, despite being prone to drink, I had a good way, so I had money to buy it. Alcohol gets you out of the way, but my goals were high. I worked hard, but that job I had also made me have a weakness for drinking, I would meet with clients and after closing the deal we would drink for hours. I could drink twenty beers a day as easily as I ate breakfast, lunch and dinner.

When you are an alcoholic you learn to fool others, this is clear, you have that gift to fool others as we fool ourselves, and when this happens we fool the one next to us. I could have several beers before going to work, nobody would notice.

I got married, for a while, I controlled my drinking, but she began to see that every day I arrived drunk from work and we talked, there, for the first time I confessed to her that I did indeed have a problem. Her words were of encouragement, we were on our way to find a solution. We started to keep track, I checked my accounts, I saw what I was spending money on, but this was no good, because at that moment I started like the man who has a lover, to hide his movements, only that the beloved woman I had, was the beer. I was laundering money so that I could buy liquor without her noticing. Sometimes with the liquor, I would get into illegal affairs, like selling things at a premium so I could keep some money to drink it.

When you get into this big hell, you don't want to talk to anybody about it, you fall into the point of being bitter, where everything is annoying, you go all day with sunglasses, hiding in your own world and looking for space for the first beer of the day. I drank and worked, nothing else, not even my wife mattered as much as she should have. In that comfort zone, I felt comfortable, where I could see and put my things. But all this left me alone, without friends, I couldn't stand anyone and I looked for solitude, drinking relaxed me, I returned to my essence. I didn't care, if the alarm went off, I would set it a little earlier so that it would give me time to have the first beer of the day.

In some moments I left my family without eating, when I got paid I took the money out of the account and I drank it all, I didn't give a damn, I drank it and already, in the hangover I regretted it a little, several times I fell into ruin, but I didn't care either, I lived in a world full of selfishness, today that causes me a lot of shame because I made many people who loved me suffer.

Today I owe money to the bank, I owe money to my family, but I have been paying this off and they understand me because they know that I went through a terrible crisis. It's six years of debt to drink, it's a lot of money.

It has been years since I tasted the first drop of liquor, for years I asked myself why, a few years ago I got the answer, as a child I had an attention deficit and I was also hyperactive, but it is something that one today when I see that my son is diagnosed with ADHD, there I analyze that I went through the same thing, but nobody treated me, the placebo was the liquor.

I always wanted to be active, but I did not know what was happening to me, I have been a doctor for a long time, the doctor sent me, but since then I have stopped the anxiety of eating, I concentrate better, I have peace of mind, I am not going to rush around the world, this multitasking thing is not for me either.

Now that I understand everything I have above, I do not suffer, I do not judge myself for what I did and did not do, I have peace in my heart, I am returning to what I was.

Of course, this was not an easy process, when I finally decided to stop drinking, I had to suffer a lot, the first time I tried, I relapsed, I tried again and it happened, here the key is not that you ask the woman you love, the child who begs you with tears or your dying mother who asks as a last will, the truth is that it has to come from within you, you have to want it, then comes the process, I fell months after entering, I tried until the fourth, where it was the defeat. I spent years without tasting a drop, but today if I drink in a meeting I do not have the desire to drink and drink, because I discovered that the root problem was not the liquor but what I wanted to cover in my emotions after the alcohol.

I remember with shame one of the times that I relapsed, I was with my people, my wife, my family, I said I was going to get water, I escaped and went to a party for three days, those three days my family looked for me until they found me asleep at a table in a bad bar.

As I said, I have to be the one who wants to stop drinking, that's how it happened before it was impossible, I remember when people told me that it was me, they stressed it so much that it sounded like a cliché, they told me that the problem was alcohol, but I had to be able to face it, I had to get to the therapies, with the double-A people, with my family, where we talked, we told each other many truths and I was realizing all my mistakes. My wife used to tell me

283

everything that I had done to her and I felt like the worst rat in the world, I didn't know that I had affected her so much, she was right in everything, it was my fault all that happened. What we were going through was curious, because she had lived one reality and I had lived another. My wife tells a thousand stories that I don't even remember, the truth is I made many mistakes.

For a while I didn't even want to smell the liquor, I prepared my meals with apple vinegar and not with wine, because they told you that if you tasted it you would fall down again, it was like you were putting to sleep the animal that wanted to drink liquor. I would see a beer and feel like throwing up, I would activate something that in my brain had been set as a red alert. It was those tools I had been given that said that with this I could eliminate the desire to drink. But the truth is that this is an anchor, living away from the vice so as not to fall, the real cure is to drink without fear of becoming an alcoholic.

Of course, this can be discussed by many, because for example, when I drank I did it in industrial quantities, alcoholism having a family is something terrible, when you thought you were fine, in fact, you were drunk, once my son had an accident, he fell and they were in the emergency room, my wife called me, I went to the hospital and she did not let me in, in fact, I was totally drunk, although I thought I was fine. My son had to be operated on and I wasn't even in the hospital because I couldn't get through.

That day, out of anger, out of spite, what I did was go to the bar, where I started drinking more until I found out that my son had come out of surgery. My wife was living like any other person, with her good and bad moments. I was on a cloud for a long time, floating and believing that I was fine. I was not.

For a long time, I lost many things, I lost my wife, my son, the relationship of trust that I had with them, even on several occasions I was violent with my wife, I raised my hand to her once, I never touched her, but I did approach her, in threat, so that she would get out of the way and leave me alone.

Until that moment, I started from scratch with my wife, I conquered her again, we went back to being the same as before and now I have worked on my emotions and I no longer live the fears of those days, that is why I can offer a Christmas without fear of missing three days or losing my mind. It's all about attitude.

Fear

As a child she loved the sights, going to those amusement parks filled with hundreds of people, buying inflated cotton, popcorn, throwing balls to try to hit the target and win the teddy bear, getting on the many sights, the wheel, the bumper cars, the roller coaster, flying chairs and other attractions full of adrenaline and fun.

Vicky loved the rides, every time her father said to go to the park, she would get so excited that she would not sleep and wait anxiously for the day until after four o'clock in the afternoon when they would go out to the park, play, ride, eat and be happy.

She would never forget the last time she set foot in an amusement park, she was thirteen years old, her father had just collected a special bonus from the company and the celebration was to enjoy to the fullest in the park, they left early, had lunch in the park and went on the rides. Normally they controlled the rides, according to the budget, this time they could ride as many times as they wanted. Vicky loved the adrenaline, she climbed the roller coaster several times, in the bumper cars she hit her companions' cars hard, and time flew by.

Although she was amused, at nightfall everything changed, she was in the flying chairs, tall, those of adults, in front of her, was a woman, she was screaming as the chair turned, Vicky was afraid that the woman would get dizzy and vomit, all that liquid would fall on her. As she turned she heard the sounds of gales, but there was a strange sound in the air, one she

286

had never heard before in the many times she had been in the chairs, it was like metals colliding.

She looked up and at the top, the screws holding the woman's chair were loose, and with the speed, it seemed to be coming off, in effect a screw came loose and held on a little longer. A couple of minutes after she realized that the chair had come loose, her screams had not been worthwhile, nor had she tried to warn of the danger, the woman was thrown up in the air, she did not see where she hit, but the attraction immediately began to stop, faster than normal.

When the view adapted, she found the woman, she had crashed into a metal post, there you could see the crack, on the ground, unconscious or dead was the woman, several people surrounded her, about 50 meters away came running some men dressed in white, apparently medical equipment.

Vicky doesn't know if the woman died or not, but because of fate it was her turn, not Vicky's, since when she got on the ride, she almost took that chair, she clearly remembers that she stood next to the chair, looked at it for an instant, saw out of the corner of her eye that the woman was coming and decided to give it to her and take the one behind her, this had been decisive in making the accident happen. If she had kept that chair she would now be injured or dead.

That day she suffered an attack, there she would know what anxiety was, they gave her to drink, hugged her and encouraged her, in the end, they had to leave, Vicky had ruined the ride, that's what her brothers said. For several days she felt guilty about the woman's accident, she bought the local newspaper looking for information about her, but nobody said anything.

Time passed, she grew up and that event apparently went to oblivion, the only thing is that that was the last time they went to that park, the attractions of this type were forgotten, now they went on excursions, to movies or to the theater. Even the invitation for their fifteenth birthday to go to Disney was not mentioned, nobody said anything, nobody missed it.

Vicky became an adult, she found a boyfriend, a loving young man who was totally seduced by her, she too was strongly attracted to him, they were in love, the young woman was already in her 24th year, she had finished a career in architecture and was about to enter a solid company with many prospects for her future.

One Saturday he wanted to surprise her, he told her he would take her to a place she would love, that would surely remind her of the past, he put her in the car and blindfolded her, drove her for a while until he reached a place where music could be heard in the distance.

The boyfriend asked her to take off the blindfold, a series of emotions came to her mind, buried in the background was the emotion of these parks, it was the first thing she remembered and on her face, a smile was drawn that her boyfriend wanted to see, but immediately she was overshadowed, she felt a tightness in her chest and saw the woman on the ground, still tied to the chair, perhaps dead. She began to tremble and her boyfriend hugged her and asked her many times what was happening.

He didn't know how to get the information out of her that day, she almost screamed at him to leave that place right now, that she couldn't be there, he took her home and the upset young woman got out without even saying goodbye.

The next day she would call him herself to talk and told him everything, the memories she had relived, he asked her for forgiveness, but she told him there was nothing to forgive.

Years later she would have to face fear, when her little daughter begged to be taken to the park, there, before riding, she checked the attraction, and what did prevent her from riding any attraction that had to do with flying chairs.

There are fears that sometimes are almost impossible to overcome.

Lack of Sleep

She's in bed again, looking at the ceiling, knowing every crack in the ceiling, she realizes that the fly from the previous night is gone, that the spider made a bigger web and it looks like she's going to live there for a while.

She has several nights looking at the ceiling and with a fear that she doesn't want to leave even though she has done everything possible not to be afraid. Hours before she was on the internet and asked how many hours can a person go without sleep to die? She was willing to never sleep again, closing her eyes and relaxing a little, but when she felt that she was going to enter the first stage of sleep she would wake up, and with this, she had already had enough days of enduring the desire to sleep and trying to never do it again.

Her company of not sleeping was weighing him down, at work she didn't perform the same, she forgot basic things like if she had eaten lunch or not, or if she had thrown soap on herself when she had bathed. She had to smell her skin to confirm that everything was okay.

She was not the same. She knew this but thought it was transitory, as she learned to live with this lack.

How did this urge not to sleep begin? It happened when she saw a horror movie, she was at night, comfortable, enjoying the film and what she thought would be a Freddie Krueger-style movie resulted in a story where people, when they slept, lost their faculties, felt that they were descending into an abyss and there they

290

were left in the darkness that did not allow them to find a way out, those who were advancing were attacked by their own fears, their insecurities and even those people who in the past marked them and now attacked with everything to make them suffer.

They never woke up again, people, in reality, remained connected in hospitals, in a coma, with no reason to know why they were sleeping, one day, the families decided to disconnect them and although the heart stopped, the minds remained alive forever, in a loop of terror in the middle of a black labyrinth with no way out.

That night, Muriel went to bed like every night, leaving the film in her subconscious, she had entertained herself and it was time to rest. As soon as she started sleeping, the same thing happened to her as to millions of people, she felt the sensation of falling and woke up from a shock, her mind immediately associated that this fall had to do with the movie, that she was on her way to go to the abyss where she would die and stay for all eternity in that world.

She started researching about it and got a website full of conspiracies, those that are so well made that they are credible, she saw the many cases of people in a coma who claimed they were in an eternal coma, to make matters worse some articles named the movie she had seen, as proof of what this evil was about and that nobody said anything, because the medical industry did not have any backing for it and did not want anyone to know because it would be a discredit, there was no research, it was just another frontier of medicine.

She joined Facebook groups where she talked to people like her who were afraid to sleep, some testimonies said that people who could not overcome sleep, fell, and dreamed, had nightmares of all kinds, it was a dystopian world, people who were persecuted by giant letters, by seas that had the waves in the opposite direction, places where the dolphins were the masters of the world, another conspiracy theory.

Many places frequently cited the film Matrix, which says that we are a simulation, so they said that when we slept and fell into those abysses we really came out of the Matrix, that we had to learn to overcome our fears to reach true freedom, there were already meditation currents to reach that nirvana, the exit from the mind. If someone in the middle of meditation, after going through some hard tests, with a body that was very hungry, thirsty, dirty, with two weeks without sleep, if he meditated and managed to reach that level, the body would stop beating, but his soul would manage to get out of the Matrix, that's why every day more and more people joined the world of non-dreaming to free themselves from these chains that had been placed on us.

There were theorists who said we were the product of reptilians, that they had put us on this farm as if we were ants and to be able to go out and be free we had to get rid of the chains of the dream, which were the moments where these beings took advantage to draw us the world that we would see the following day.

Not to sleep is freedom. They said some of the phrases that people created.

292

That's why Muriel was determined never to sleep a wink again, she drank industrial quantities of coffee, every day she served herself a generous cup that she drank in long, heavy sips to wake up a drunk. Although she had big dark circles under her eyes and each one of her muscles hurt, she continued to endure, thinking that this would be like the ketogenic diet, the first step was the hardest, educating the body to consume energy from fat and not from carbohydrates, which when passing the threshold, could live not sleeping, just closing her eyes for a while and resting or in a superficial meditation where the organs rested and the body was put in a rest that regenerated them. Many in this type of meditation fell asleep, but the goal was to rest and to be able to continue. This far from being a meditation was a short sleep.

Muriel began to meditate and try to rest the body, while she controlled her breathing, her mind began to see unknown images, she got up, she had fallen asleep for five minutes, she felt the same tiredness, she closed her eyes again and entered the non-dream phase, where the body rested. His goal was to meditate until he reached the level of leaving the body and getting out of the Matrix or escaping from the reptilians who wanted to control us in the ant farm.

About a fortnight her boss called her at the office and handed her a check that had more money in it than she normally got, much more, he told her that there was her paycheck for her fortnight and the settlement, that she could not return that she could not have an employee who spent the day sleeping or nodding off and trying not to stay in the chair without attending to

293

the work, that her quality of work had been lost by 80%.

She thought she was not sleeping, but apparently, she had gone so many days without sleep because during the day she would fall asleep for a few seconds every now and then. Her boss showed her the recordings and there she was, after two o'clock in the afternoon, lowering her head and falling asleep for a while. In the recording they showed her, she was like this for ten minutes, then she lifted her head up and continued working, but apparently, she did that several times a day.

She had to look for a solution to not sleep, she would fall into the abyss, she would stay in the infinite hell from which she would never come out again and God knew that if she fell there she would meet many people she had left behind who wanted to hurt her and remind her of monsters she had left behind.

She devoted herself to read more, to investigate, she met a shaman who lived in the city and had a meditation center, he charged an inscription of 5 thousand dollars, but he promised that she would always get out of that bad habit of sleeping, she did not doubt it, she had money from the liquidation of the company, she went there and received material, characters that had never slept after discovering this, from beings that one day were here and the next day disappeared, that managed to transcend.

Sure that she was entering the path she deserved, she went to the first class with the shaman. There were dozens of people, just like her, all with dark circles under their eyes, exhausted, but with a bitter smile and hope, promising themselves that they would come out of this, that they would transcend in order to live without the vice of sleep.

The shaman helped them with a type of meditation based on mantras and with high caffeine drinks to keep them awake. The one who fell asleep was awakened with loud noises of dishes, which made them awake and helped the others who were in the process of falling asleep.

After the initiation meditation, they would go to meditate with dances, rhythmic movements that kept them active. The shaman recommended to be always active, doing some task, he recommended not to read, to see movies or to lie down to rest, the bed was not an object of first necessity, they even had to pick it up, they had to stand up and when they sat down they had to do it in hard chairs.

One day, Muriel went to see the shaman tell him that she was managing not to sleep and to feel lucid, that she was thinking better, that she was surely reaching the level of freedom. When she opened the door, the shaman, the old man with the white beard, was on a delicious white bed, padded with three pillows and sleeping like a cat, without any concern.

There, as if a great truth was revealed, all the images of the last months came to Muriel's mind and she discovered that she was playing the role of an idiot. The shaman got wise and was going to explain to her what was happening, but she didn't give him time, she left that place and went home.

She slept for three days straight.

Living with Bipolar

Theresa and Basil are husbands, she took her husband for a long time as a volatile person, someone who at any stimulus could jump out of anger, but as he gets older, his symptoms seem worse.

She has always been afraid to say anything to her husband because when he talks to her, she expects him to respond in a good, neutral way or with a violence that is not relevant, although sometimes he also responds with a euphoria that is not understood.

Some time ago he was diagnosed with bipolarity and this explained many things, she did not understand that her husband was so strange, despite knowing the consequences of what he had, this did not diminish the importance of what happened, she lived in fear, guilt and tried many times not to talk to Basil, because she expected any bad reaction. Even though he went into treatment, there was no shortage of days when she was abused, when she was again the victim of his attacks.

Basil loves his wife, he is clear about this and has shown it to her many times, although sometimes it is inevitable that he does not act against her and shows her a side that even he is afraid of. Some believe that sometimes he is happy, he goes through euphoria, but in reality, he feels this when he has irritability, anger that he cannot control, and manic desires to end everything. He has felt that his life can be an attempt against others and against himself.

One of the reasons why he sometimes looked bad, was because he was in periods of mania, hypomania, sometimes looked depressed, passed several times from one state to another and to healthy means, that is, he was sometimes full of much joy, and sometimes with depression, all with his face not showing it, but with strong desires to express it.

My doctor has told me that one of the best ways is for me to retire, take breaks, eat well and exercise, and of course, medicate myself, but the truth is that I do not want to exercise and rest at night, because during the day I have work, the medicine is always given to me by my wife.

A few days ago my wife was fighting me, complaining because I was spending some money, I wanted to buy that ornament, even though I had one in the living room, but my wish was to have it in the room, to have two, I do not see anything wrong with that, but she fought me and told me that that money was to pay the rent, that I could not take that money, she shouted at me, I got upset and for a change, we ended up holding on the street, in a strong argument where everybody was a witness, it is not the first time, nor will it be the last. Very common among us is this kind of a mess.

Sometimes it is difficult for me to bear with Basil, I have to understand that sometimes it is difficult for him to understand the subject of money, that he does not understand the responsibility of it. But I know that he does when he goes through the moments of hypomania and then comes out with the depression because we have to resolve with the money to pay and he has to borrow on many occasions.

When he suffers the episodes of bipolarity, the episodes of anxiety appear, where he shows himself worse, combining the condition, he sweats, blows the bag like a TV character, breathes in and out, strongly, and cannot bear to be with himself, in those moments, although it breaks my heart to see him so badly, I leave him alone, not to get hurt because I understand that to go to him, to tell him that he will get out of this, is to see his worst face emerge and to say that it is easy for me to say empty words, that I am a fool, that what a mistake he made in picking on me and that I wish he suffered from the same so that he would know that the words "morons" don't fit me.

I know that this disease I suffer from has no cure, that there are many studies, but the truth is there is no cause for bipolar disorder and from the genetics of the brain structure, the effort to better understand this has its advances, but they are not as important as I would like. There are medications, there are therapies, to help us, but surely we will have to take them until we die.

The worst thing of all is that it could get worse, it is my worst fear, right now I am a very functional person, but always being that there is something spying in the corner that could undo that.

In case you have experienced a manic episode, I can guarantee you that another one will come, that psychosis is a key part of the bipolar process, and that when it happens we lose contact with reality at some point in our existence. I was once hospitalized for depression, and although I haven't been, I have found suicide to be an extremely seductive way out. My doctor agrees with me, my disorder can get worse, but if I take my medication and follow the guidelines I will be able to keep myself under control. So he says.

Sometimes I stop being me, it's frustrating to put it simply. I suffer from very strong headaches, and sometimes I get asthma, it's something that goes with me, hand in hand, I don't always have a headache, fortunately, but I have to put up with bipolar disorders and that's every day, all the time.

Even when the symptoms are kept in control, I have to do constant monitoring, I have to do it, and I keep doing it so that an episode doesn't go off, when depression appears, you have to fight so that control is not lost, I do it many times.

I am manic, I get irritated easily and sometimes I am not as competent as I would like, I get depressed, I get filled with fears and even some voices in my head that try to distort reality and I start to question the feelings I have had, the actions I have taken.

In all this type with Basil I have spent incredible moments and some where I have been complicated, he has had seasons of lows, where he gets very depressed and others where he has been well, happy and moving. In the bad ones, it's time to push him, to help him reach the goal.

When he has highs, it seems that he eats up the world, that he can handle everything, that he wanted more of everything, even more sex, and to work a lot, to do many things, everything but sleep, he didn't need it, in those highs I felt outside, as if he only cared about... him.

Suffering from bipolar disorder is like being on a roller coaster full of many emotions, sometimes you're on top and sometimes you fall hard against a wall. Relationships get complicated, and if we add the part that everything can get complex, then there are relationships with the disorder that make you suffer wherever you look.

When a bipolar person is in the depressive phase, it is necessary to treat him/her as if he/she were a depressive. When he gets euphoric, I help him, although the first time I thought he was on drugs, because he wasn't and suddenly he acts that way, I told myself he had smoked a joint.

It was hard for me to understand that this was not the fault of his education, of his roots, but that it was genetic or stress or the person, not what he lived as a child, so I took the blame away from the mother, it's not the fault of that poor woman.

Recently they took Basil to the hospital because he was very euphoric, worse than ever, he wanted to do tasks from which he could later get hurt, and he could not afford it. Many of the treatments they give him can help him get back to normal. It hurts me to have him taken away like a madman, but it's the only way I can help him recover.

Again I'm in this crazy place, I'm not crazy, I'm not, I don't know when they will understand, my wife doesn't understand, I'm not crazy, I just have bipolarity. They tell me that I am not crazy, that they only take care of me and they expect me to calm down so that I don't do anything that threatens me, that when I calm down I will return home, that's what they say, that's what I expect them to do because if not, I don't know what I will do. I'm not crazy, I'm not...

The Arrival of the Red Submarine

I am not a man who has had many women in life, I had some, as a young man in school I dated some, in graduation I had my moment of sex with the girl I liked and nothing formal, at least until I came of age, when I had my first girlfriend, with more mistakes than successes, fights and learning to have a girlfriend, those relationships undoubtedly ended. What was left was my experience to start having more solid relationships, the first ways, while I was forging myself as a professional and as a man.

During this time I understood about women who had good moments and bad moments that sometimes they were in a bad mood and could not stand each other and other times they were happy and wanted everything. On certain days of the month, I would tell myself that her belly was hurting, that she was in a bad mood, nothing out of the ordinary in what one expects with a woman.

Finally, I fell in love, Rose is the woman who stole my heart, she appeared like a whirlwind with all her good energy and I don't know how to explain it, but I got hooked on her, she was everything I always looked for in a woman, with her I felt that I was where I always wanted to be, it seems she also started to feel the same, because we were always together, sharing and happy, completely in love. We married for everything: for the civil, the church, and for idiots. We began to live together and the first weeks were the best, as expected of any newlywed relationship, but soon I began to notice that something was happening, the first time it was not so accentuated, she was crying in the corners and telling me that everything was fine, but she spent practically the whole day crying as if someone had died, she told me that the days of her menstrual period were a little sad ... I did not want to imagine what would be a time of hostility, it would be worse.

For several months, we were close and everything seemed to be going well, except for those two-day-a-month episodes where she was crying, but when the relationship settled down a bit, the rules of the game changed. One morning when I woke up I found her standing in the kitchen, looking at the faucet, the water was running and she had some dishes in her hands.

When I went to see her, to see if she was all right, to dry her tears, that was what I was waiting for, she already had the rhythm of her cycle, but she looked at me with hate like she had never done before.

—Am I your servant woman?

—What are you talking about love? —Are you all right?

—I'm not, how can I be when my father paid for me to go to college and end up living in the house with a man who asks me to make him breakfast, to take care of him, the king! I have to serve the king the delicacies, oh and he probably wants sex, because how he loves it when I make him moan. Is that what I am to you? A woman of service and the whore who is your wife. Is that why we got married?

—Love! If it's about making breakfast, go ahead, go to bed, sit down and talk while I prepare it, of course not, you know I like to cook, if on Sundays you eat my pancakes.

—You send me to sit down because you consider me the useless one of the house, that I cannot even prepare your breakfast, is that it?

—Not at all, I woke up happy, I came to greet you, you are the one who fights with me

—Then I am a bitter one.

—Well, right now you are. Quite so, you've never been like that with me

—This is me! If you don't like it, then fuck you, because I won't change, that's me, this is the one you married, the one you have chained to cook and give you sex.

—I don't understand you.

—I'm clear about that, you don't understand me at all, nobody understands me, what a misfortune, not even my husband understands me, for you, I'm just a mannequin, a useless creature.

—Love, but you seem to be crazy.

—"Yes, I am a madwoman," she began to cry, —that's what I am to you, a stupid madwoman.

She said this and went to her room, locked herself in, and cried all morning, the pleas I made to her were not answered, and finally, I went to prepare breakfast.

Around one o'clock in the afternoon, she came out, crying, walking softly, with her hands held, looking at me with guilt.

—Forgive me, I'm a fool, I got my period, I'm sick, you know I don't take it well. That sometimes I get a little hostile.

—You scared me, love.

—Sometimes I get like this a little before it gets to me, but as soon as it appears I get well, well, a little sad, but everything else passes, I'm fine now, do you forgive me?

I had no other choice, I went to hug her and we talked, deep down I felt a bad feeling, I couldn't stand her being like that, having that meaningless hostility, suddenly being the sweetest, the one I fell in love with and then behaving like a crazy person.

They say that when you get married you really start to get to know your partner, I was already starting to get to know her and I didn't like it, I wasn't attracted to the way my wife behaved and I was afraid, I don't know what could happen the next month.

I would have to be prepared. After this scene I downloaded an application to my cell phone and started counting the days, when the pink squares were there, thinking that soon the hostility would appear again.

One morning I found it in the kitchen, this time it was not hostile, but I was afraid. I saw her hand on my chest, she was looking at me with fear, I ran to her side, fearing that she might be having a heart attack, she was breathing heavily, smiling and putting her hand on my arm, but she was running to the bathroom and spitting up, she was in a picture of anxiety.

—How did love help you?

—Hold me.

I did...

—No, no, let go, I can't, sorry, I can't. I'm so scared.

—But why? Something happened.

—No, never, I'm just very afraid, just stay with me.

I stood by her side, while she was suffering, with her face unraveled, breathing heavily, with a fear that came from within her and she did not know how to control it. A couple of times she got up to vomit, the second time she told me.

—You see me vomiting and you don't even hold my hair.

I get up to help her, but she told me what for, that I don't need it anymore. She goes to her room, still anxious, but now also angry.

All the women I've gone out with have never behaved so unhinged, she had something I'd never seen before.

Hours later the scene of last month was repeated, she was in her day, we had already overcome the scene of the month.

The next month I met her again in the kitchen, she had the big knife in her hand, the one for chopping meat, she was holding it over her wrist. I ran and took the knife away from her.

—Why are you doing that? You can't kill yourself.

—"I'm just so sad," she said and began to cry more.

I hugged her and this month we were lucky because after a while she got back to normal.

The next month I found her eating, she was euphoric, but she ate everything, she had a cake that we had bought the day before and she ate it with a lot of anxiety and invited me to try it with her, that month was not so bad, we shared and my anxiety to know what she would have this time passed.

It also happened that when I presented the problems with her period, I began to live anchored in it, I was always worried about what could happen to her, the behaviors I might have, so instead of enjoying my recent marriage, I was only worried about waiting for the scene of the next month.

I decided to start taking control of the situation, I opened the internet and started searching, everywhere they talked about the bad mood and other details of the month, illnesses, situations, complications, and sanitary pads, there seemed to be no reason for her to behave like that, when I was about to give up and think with regret that my wife was simply crazy, I found a disease that coincided perfectly with her: premenstrual dysphoric disorder.

I kept digging into that subject and it seemed to describe my wife and that worried me, I would have to wait at least until menopause for her to stop committing these crazy things.

The recommendations I found were to eat healthy, exercise, keep a diary of what happens every month, I already have that, reduce salt, sugar, caffeine, help her sleep better, yes, I saw how hard it was for her to sleep every night.

I waited a week for her period to pass so I could talk about what I had read.

—I think I know what you have.

—"I have nothing," she says, —what are you talking about?

—Your behavior every time you get your period.

—All women get a little bitter when it comes.

—Yours is epic.

—Now you know women better than women. It's normal.

—You wanted to kill yourself!

—It was a picture of anxiety, that's all, I'm great.

—You have a disorder, it's called the premenstrual dysphoric disorder

—What a great invention that is. You are insane.

There was no way, that day we ended up arguing and I got angry because I had taken the trouble to talk to her, to tell her what was going on and I turned out to be a villain. So what I decided to do was to leave her alone and start researching more, I found out that antidepressants could help, so before her period arrived I served her coffee and put her on antidepressants.

For a few months it worked, she was happy, but one morning she found me crushing the pills in her cup, we had a serious fight and she did not receive any more food. The next month the episodes, fights, suicide attempts, anger, depression returned. My patience was already exhausted because I wanted to help but she wouldn't let me, so I approached her and we started to fight more, in her sad days I would say some strong things to her and she would cry, in the months of anger, the fights seemed endless, as if we hated each other. We began to spend days without speaking to each other or sleeping in the same bed.

This is the day where there is still no solution, I don't know what will happen next month, but my hopes are placed on her to listen to me and to commit herself to treat her condition, to see if we can find harmony in this home.

I miss my wife, the one I fell in love with, who never seemed to get her period, not this one, who explodes every month.

The calendar on my cell phone tells me that she'll get it any minute, so we'll see what kind of surprise this month brings.

Thanksgiving Day

They didn't talk to each other, as happens with many couples who can go a long time without speaking, they didn't speak at all, they didn't talk, they didn't say a supportive or fighting sentence to each other, they were simply two strangers sharing a roof.

It may be a bit curious to be in a marriage where the couple hasn't spoken to each other for years, but in the Thompsons, this had been going on for twenty years, the comedians who made jokes about marriages surely were inspired by them to create their themes.

Their children got used to seeing them not talking, not sharing anything with each other, and sleeping in different rooms.

The reader will wonder how they communicated the topics about the home, about care, shopping, medicine for a child, paying for school, everything, over the years they communicated through third parties, mostly with the children, and always told with love.

—Son, tell your dad that the food is served.

The little one would go for his father and he would come to eat, in silence, when he finished, without his wife listening, he would tell the son:

—Tell your mother that the food was very good, but that the avocado was very salty, and that tomorrow I would like to eat some ribs.

311

The son was obedient to tell his mother what he had told him, so over the years, they communicated everything.

The children grew up, they left home and the two old men were left alone, here the communication became a little more difficult, but they knew how to communicate, as expected, the idea came from the woman, who prepared a leaf and put it on the door of the refrigerator.

—I've left a notebook on the table, we can write to each other here, breakfast is covered, when you want to eat it, you serve it to yourself. Enjoy your meal.

The man ate and left his first note next to the plate.

The couple had years without speaking, although some nights, not so much now, the man visited her bed, got in, caressed her back, she looked at him and ran the sheet, got in and they loved each other in silence, as soon as their breaths gave notice that they were in the midst of pleasure, in the end, they finished, the man got dressed and as soon as he arrived he slipped into her bed.

Something about the woman was that she had an unbreakable word, when she was young she started smoking, she did it for a couple of years, she would light a cigarette with the previous one. One day, she got a bad case of pneumonia, the doctor told her it was the fault of the two packs of cigarettes she smoked a day. Then, she stopped, quit smoking, told her husband, at the time she was talking to him, that she would never smoke a cigarette again, that's right, she never tried it again, everyone doesn't know if she would suffer from abstinence, but her word was kept.

Her children were afraid of her because they knew very soon that she did not threaten in vain, if she told you that if you continued with that attitude you would not go out for that walk, be sure that you would not go out, that you would be punished, if she told you that she was going to hit you with the strap, it was not a threat, it was a notification.

Just as she was rigid, she was also sweet and loved festivities, for example, on birthdays she loved to enjoy herself, when her husband had his birthday, she would leave a gift next to him in bed. Usually, it was something he liked, something he needed. Even if she didn't talk to him, she would leave his present on the spot.

But of all the holidays, the one she loved most was Thanksgiving, it was magic for her, she would start preparing it two months before and she always wanted to have the family together. That day, because it was special, was an exception, the spouses talked to each other, it was the only day they talked all year round.

When he would get up she would receive him with a smile, like the best wife, she would look at him and tell him with a love as if they had spoken the day before.

—Last night I prepared your clothes for today, I'm going to make you breakfast. Eggs or bacon?

—You know, bacon, I love it.

—As my man says.

313

She prepared the food, the woman that day, when she put the plate next to him, gave him a kiss on the cheek or a little kiss on the mouth. They were the happy family, during the day, at night, the family would start arriving, they would have an incredible evening, they would drink, eat and be so full that they would open their pants. In the end, the whole family would leave, and only they, a few years later the children, would be left alone. They would pick up everything, talk about the evening, and when they finished picking up everything, she would take his hand and they would go to their room, make love like they hadn't done all year, with passion, whispering dirty words to each other and reaching orgasm with the pleasure that the already established couple is known for.

At twelve o'clock at night, the charm was broken, he got up, went to his bed, and returned to the same hermeticism of always.

How did this happen?

For years the couple talked without a problem, but one time, the husband slipped up with his assistant at the office, it was only a one afternoon stand, but since he was not very professional in these deception deals, he committed the brutality of leaving the motel receipt in his pants pocket.

The woman found it, approached him, had the typical fight one would expect after a betrayal, and threw away the sentence, she said:

—From this moment on, I will never speak to you again, this will be the last conversation that you and I will ever have

—Love, but this is not for you to act like this.

—I'm not leaving you because we have three children, because I don't want them to grow up without a father as I did. That's why we'll stay in this house and not fight and not try to have scenes and hate in front of them, this house is as much yours as it is mine, so when they grow up, we'll still be here, but we'll never talk again.

—That seems a little radical to me.

—We only talk one day a year and because that day is important to me, Thanksgiving.

The man took the woman's reaction as crazy, he thought it would be an outburst of anger, but let's remember that she had a word and she made it count, she didn't speak to him again, at first she ignored him, he spoke to her in a thousand ways, but the woman didn't listen, sometimes he sent her a folded piece of paper with one of his children saying

—Don't talk to me, I told you, on Thanksgiving we talked, but not about this, I hate fighting that day. Everything is clear now, don't talk to me, you're overwhelming me.

The man tried for months to get a word out of the woman, but she did not give in, finally, she gave in and on the first Thanksgiving day she spoke to him as if nothing had happened, they made love and with three minutes to go before twelve she said.

—It will be time, we'll talk in a year, get out of my bed.

The man insisted, he spoke, but at twelve o'clock at night, the woman fell into silence. 365 days of silence.

In the end, she got used to it, it was her habitat, to get used to it or to leave it, and the latter was not in question.

Her children, when they became conscious, began to wonder why their parents were not speaking to each other, when they asked the father this one with bitterness he said to ask the mother when they asked her she said to ask the father what he had done.

Years later, they learned that because of a fight the woman had sentenced him not to talk to her anymore. They already knew the woman's character, so it didn't surprise them.

When the husband was sick, she would attend to him, go to his room and place the medicine on the night table with a note of the amount to be taken. She did not ask him if he had taken the dose but checked either the spoon or the bottle to confirm that he had indeed taken the medicine.

On other days, when she was sick, he would come by, take care of her, and say things to her with words, worrying about her, forgetting the pact they had. The woman ignored him but followed the instructions.

Eventually, old age caught up with them, the woman did not speak, not even when she heard about his stomach cancer, she would go to his side for consultations, ask the doctor about his doubts and they would return home, on the days of chemotherapy she would stay by his side, when she threw up she would help him clean up, she was an impeccable nurse, she never complained, never asked, she seemed to know everything.

The man finally died, not on a day of grace, but in the middle of the year. On the coffin was the woman leaning, watching him rest, with a sad face.

When they finally closed it to bury him, she said in a broken voice.

—Oh, my old man.

She cried and lamented for the first time the silence of so many years.

The Habit

Holly and Bolton have been married for several years. How does a couple get used to doing the same thing over and over again without wanting to kill each other?

They met one night in a bar, they were the roll of a Friday, two unknown people, they liked each other, they understood each other in bed and the next day they each went on with their lives. They said that they had nothing more to say to each other, that they had to get on with their lives and that this was just a one-night stand, they both agreed and both forgot

About a month later they met again in a bar, they talked and felt a different vibration, the two had desires for each other, and they found themselves in bed again, wishing each other, wanting to have sex, at dawn they said goodbye again forever, saying that it had been an exception to the rule

The point is that they kept meeting, they kept seeing each other and they liked each other more and more and the sexual encounters were more intense.

Soon they got into the habit of having these encounters, even though they said they lived somewhat sporadically, the encounter took place in a bar, they ended up in the same hotel, and repeated the same movements in bed, they even got to a point of having the same room, they already knew the scars on the walls and the sounds in the mattress, the trick of the key when opening and the exact point to make it warm as they liked, they knew the steps that separated the

318

door of the room from the ice machine and the time when the maid spent the next day collecting the dirt and cleaning rooms.

They made a habit of doing the same thing and repeated it. One day, they began to get tired of these supposedly accidental encounters, and scheduled a date outside the party environment, invited her to dinner. They went to a fish place, where they ate some sea paella that they both liked with a white wine recommended by the chef, they got to know each other better, she was aspiring to be an actress, he was composing songs and selling them to different musicians, her wish was that one of those lyrics would be bought by some famous singer.

There was romance in the air, they already knew each other's skins and knew they understood each other well, although until then they were a bit drunk. That night, after dinner, they went to a better hotel, one that did not have the walls so thin as to filter the sound from the neighboring rooms.

With a bed that had no sound and a TV that had more than porn channels. For the first time, they made love with romance, they carefully walked around giving each other pleasure, fell asleep hugging like an old married couple, kissed at dawn, and made love in the shower.

They ordered breakfast from the room and continued the encounter for many more hours, walking unhurriedly, discovering each other, and giving way to what would be a nascent relationship. Soon they were formal boyfriends, and the meetings were not so common in a hotel, but began to go to galleries, concerts, he received her in the failed auditions that were all, never called, some were deceptive offers to work as a prostitute and encouraged her when she decided to start working in a cafe.

On Mondays, they did not see each other because he went to an event, on Tuesdays they met after seven o'clock when she left work, on Wednesdays it was repeated, on Thursdays they did not see each other because it was the night where she met with other failed actors, on Fridays they met and spent the weekend at his house, eating pizza, reheated food and watching series on shift. Two years passed in this cycle, repeating the ritual without changes except for extraordinary exceptions.

After a fight, on her part, because she was tired of the same thing, he solved everything with an engagement ring, which was kept for a year and a half by more than one engaged couple to be able to step up to the altar.

Another fight put a date on it, now, the happy couple was on the same roof, with the same bills and the commitments. She wanted children, but he was not prepared, two years went by and many fights to make them take the step and start making love in every corner to be able to get pregnant.

Six months later, she was given the miracle, she had a delay, they bought a pregnancy test and it was positive, nine months later a little boy was born who changed the dynamics of the home, and the custom began to fall apart, they did not do so much the same things, but tried new experiences.

As the child grew, they tried other things, but when the little one reached seven years of age everything returned to the routine, the man came home from work and started watching television, he did not share with the little one, the latter asked him to play, to do new things, but he did not attend to him, his mother did not attend to him either, she was on her cell phone, complaining about her husband who did not attend to the child or to her.

They say you become the person you surround yourself with, Holly was, a female version of her husband, now she was living in the same cycle of routines, of procrastinating and doing the same thing over and over again. The boy reached adolescence, built his world, and walked with his friends, except to get to sleep, the young man was never at home.

Married, immersed in routine, everything seemed normal to him, they lived at their own pace, doing their own things, each one living in the routines. They had already established them, she did the chores, he put the food on, watched TV and talked a little about work, he had given up music, he was frustrated like Holly who was never an actress.

Without fail, every Saturday night, he would caress her, kiss her and repeat the same route, putting his hand through some folds, running his tongue through others, opening with his fingers, entering, giving himself the same amount of movements, she would have a mechanical orgasm or sometimes she would fake it and he would finish soon after, she would wash and he would wipe himself with paper.

321

They would watch TV as if nothing had happened, half an hour later he would fall asleep and she would change and put on some channel that she liked, when she was sleepy she would fall asleep and so on until Sunday, when he would wake up after ten o'clock, she had already made breakfast, had lunch on the way and the house was clean.

She would read the newspaper, while she was having breakfast, the time would be tied up with lunch, when she ate, they would go to bed to watch some series together, take naps, drink coffee and the routine of the week would start on Monday, until Friday again.

It was a routine of years that although it seemed that neither of them cared, it was already boring, he did not care about her, if they asked him he would realize that he did not care much, he did not love her, if she was missing the only thing he would miss would be the habit of seeing her there.

She loved him, but since she had a lot of love, she was immensely bored by the man, thinking about him made her want to yawn, she knew what he was going to say, she could almost imitate him because every sentence he said on every day of the week she knew by heart, sometimes she was ahead of what he was going to ask because she already knew he would ask.

Whoever has never been married could say that this marriage was doomed to failure, but no, it was the typical American marriage and from many parts of the world, eternal couples who were stuck in their own comfort zones and even though they were extremely boring they felt at ease.

322

Old age caught up with them and with it the routines, with age people acquire strange customs, old manias, they called it. She got used to being with the man with his accidental farts, he had gotten used to a woman who gave hostile answers, the product of the age that allowed him not to shut up at all.

The two would die together, one would die first than the other, their son would come every now and then to visit them, bringing them food, because they no longer worked, now with them at home all the time, the habits were more intense, the customs were more accentuated. He watched TV all day, took a dog they had out for a walk, fed the pigeons in a park, and, like an old cat, slept all afternoon.

Arranging socks, arranging clothes, and looking for what to do, the habit of being active prevented her from living the lazy life her husband had. As for the two of them, they could spend the whole day close by, next to each other, and not talk, not because they were angry at all, but because they were used to their presence.

And after so many years of marriage, there is not much to say to each other, and when they do not do anything transcendental, they do not have much to say to each other, except that a dove shat the dog, or that the dog beat the buttock of a child, or she hurt her thumb with a needle, or that the grinder locked again.

Habits are the best glue for eternal love.

The Bed

Daryl was married, he had a wife with whom he had lived for fifteen years, an ordinary marriage that doesn't deserve many lines, because you would yawn from boredom. The relationship already had so many cracks that he had chosen to have one of those lovers who behaves like girlfriends and does everything that regular women don't. In exchange, he gave her what she needed, money for her expenses, the rent for the cell phone, the house and to buy her cleaning supplies.

His lover was a 19-year-old white girl with pink lips, thin and contoured legs, a beautiful body with round breasts and small nipples, who would hump when she made love and do what no one else had done to her that purred like no other that had him in love lusting after that woman with intensity.

Every Wednesday, he would tell his mother that he would go bowling and go to the small apartment he had with his lover and they would make love, eat, talk and behave like a couple of boyfriends. Daryl was getting younger with Crystal, looking forward to that day every week.

The relationship could have continued without the setbacks, if something hadn't started happening in his life. On one visit while he was in bed with her, he felt warmer than usual, even though he had just gone to bed. Normally, when you first lie down in bed, you feel the cloth cold, at room temperature, but soon, the body heat makes it warm. When a person lies down on a bed that has just been vacated, it feels warm, the residual heat of the body. That's what he felt that first time.

He didn't say anything, at that moment he had Crystal undressing and devouring him with kisses, but days later, already calm, he began to think about Crystal's bed, to make conjectures about what could be happening, tying up loose ends, thinking about if under the bed could have been a naked man listening to what she was saying in the midst of the passion she considered her girlfriend. For his own sanity, he preferred to think that everything had been the object of his insecurity.

Many nights, when his wife was sleeping and he heard her soft snoring, and he took the opportunity to use his cell phone, but also to write to Crystal, he usually answered her immediately and they talked for a long time, what every lover says, words of love, hot conversations, some pictures of her, to put it, telling her he wanted it. There were days when she would write him hot messages, with pictures, make up a whole hot story and then, when she had it melted, ask him for something. She was no saint, she knew how to get anything from her man.

The following Wednesday, he went to see her, he had in his unconscious the idea of the bed, from the living room while they were talking he saw it out of the corner of his eye, he even detailed it underneath, it was empty, they talked, kissed, had dinner and went to bed, when she sat down she felt him warm, I could say even warmer than the previous week. He said nothing, but felt uncomfortable the whole encounter because he could not enjoy his beloved. Many theories were going through his head about what could be the reason for that bed to be warm.

The question became more critical, because as the weeks went by the bed became hotter and hotter, to the point that one night he found it so hot that it was difficult to get into it.

—What's wrong, love? Come to bed, this kitten is waiting for you.

The woman would wiggle around half-naked and ask him to get into bed. The man did not want to give in, the temptation was great, but he was eager to know what was happening.

—This bed is on fire.

—Of course, if I'm in it, it's on fire, waiting for you.

—No, it's not that, it's literally hot.

—I don't understand you.

—The bed, touch it, it's hot.

Crystal touched, raised her shoulders as if to imply that she was normal.

—Every week I sell I feel the bed getting hotter, right now it's about to burn, I don't know how you're standing on it.

—Love, have you gone crazy? Every week I wait anxiously for you and now that I'm here, all for you, you go crazy.

She said that and opened her legs, showing her panty and inviting him to come, Daryl took her, lifted her and placed her on the couch in the living room, they made love there, she felt excited because they were trying new things, doing it in other places, he forgot for a while that he had left the bed because it was burning without knowing for what reason.

When they finished, they went to take a bath, when they went out, without her noticing, she touched the bed and it was cold, it was as if no one had been in it all day.

He didn't understand what was going on, but this put him in a bad mood, because he knew that something was hiding behind this situation, the woman could be hiding something or he was going crazy.

That week he was in a bad mood, thinking the worst, when she didn't immediately respond to his messages he imagined the worst that Crystal was with another man in bed, that he had his turn on Wednesdays and everyone had their turn to be with her. The bad mood was unbearable, he fought with his wife a couple of times, all because of him, who responded badly to the woman's comments.

At work, he was in a bad mood, his subordinates couldn't stand him, they were afraid to even talk to him. When he arrived on Wednesday, he arrived a little earlier at her house, but he did not get out of the car, but stayed there watching, after a while, he realized that the woman was not hiding anything, he even wrote her a message that where he was then he got out, entered the house and shared with her, the bed was

327

warm again, not burning like the previous week, but it seemed to have been occupied. They made love, ordered pizza, and that night, for the first time in their lives, he slept with her, it wasn't planned, they were hugging, talking, one was silent, then the other and they fell asleep.

The next day, at six o'clock in the morning, he went home quickly, his wife would surely be furious, what would be his surprise when he arrived, she greeted him as if nothing had happened and went to sleep for a while, then she bathed, went to work and his wife did not even bother to ask him where he had spent the night.

The suspicions with Crystal did not end, one night, not Wednesday, he went to her house, parked half a block away, and dedicated himself to observe, attentive to see if anything happened, the house was quiet, nobody went out, nobody entered. The next day he did the same thing, only this time he got off and went over to the house, tried to listen, looked behind the curtain, saw her pass by, into the kitchen, she looked lonely. Even the day he saw her pass by with her cell phone in her hand, he jumped up and down, because at the moment he wrote to her, the woman seemed to be open only to him.

Other nights he went to visit her, they shared and continued their eternal romance with a beautiful spring. Daryl decided one day to do something risky, he called her and told her to get ready, that he would go get her, it was a Friday, he was already waiting for her outside the house, but she didn't say anything, he had her tested. The woman left on time, beautiful as ever, they went to dinner and returned, that night again he stayed with her at home, the next morning, this time without worrying about the woman's reaction, he arrived at mid-morning, it was Saturday, so he settled in his bed and slept all day. His wife didn't even claim him.

The encounters continued and Crystal's bed was still warm, but it hadn't gotten as hot as it had weeks before. Although he watched her, he never saw another man in her house and everything she said seemed to be real, he didn't pretend to hide anything and the lover's relationship that now moved on to something more formal, seemed not to displease him, on the contrary, he seemed at ease.

One day, the bed simply stopped being warm, it was as if this whole episode had never happened, by chance it started to be normal when he fell more in love with Crystal and wanted to live with her, to share his life with that young woman. He took the step, he didn't care, he was even determined to send his wife to hell. He was considering asking her for a divorce, it would be the best thing to do to move to Crystal's house for good.

The day he proposed it to his lover, she was thrilled, she liked the idea of having him there every day, not sleeping alone every night. She had also not been indifferent to the attachment they had had in recent times, so she gladly accepted.

Daryl stayed at her house, the next day he arrived home, ready to talk to his wife, she didn't ask him where he was, he took a bath, changed and went out to look for his wife, he couldn't find her, he missed her going out, he went into the bedroom, checked the closet and saw that she had put on the dress she used for special dates, one he had given her years ago, it was a signature dress and it looked beautiful.

She missed it, but she didn't give it much thought, she went to bed, as soon as she sat down on it, she had to get up, it was burning, like embers, she put her hand twenty centimeters closer and felt the steam in her palm.

Sometimes the games are mutual.

The Infinite Thread of Drinks

After leaving work he walked to the street where he usually walked. He knew every inch of that place, although he hadn't stepped on it for fifteen years. There he stayed, looking at his premises, seeing that time had not passed through them, although the faces he saw were new, deciding whether to go home or stay there, he had needed to come to this street for quite some time.

He walked to the place he had always visited, he knew it well, he stopped at the door and detailed it, there are countless times he left there totally drunk, he sighed, he knew he had no choice, so he went in. The interior of the place was also identical to how he remembered it, the usual bad-smelling tables, the people sitting there drinking and thinking about their things, some happy playing dominoes, others talking at full speed and at the back the bar, where their hunched backs drank slowly. He went and took the chair that was available, sat down, and looked at the man who was attending, it took him several seconds to recognize him, he was the same barman as always, grayer, with more belly and wrinkles.

The man looked at him, contemplated for a while that face that was familiar to him, but he also had more wrinkles and weight.

—Collins? —he asked. —The same, and as handsome as ever.

—I thought I'd never see you again.

—You see. Give me the usual.

The man, as if he had just seen him the day before, walked over, took the bottle of white rum, and poured the first drink of the night into his glass.

In another life, Collins never left this place. Every night when he finished work, he would come to the bar and his dinner would be rum until he felt his head spinning, walked home, went to bed, and stood up when the alarm clock was beating his head. He could have been like that all his life, with a permanent hangover and poor nutrition, if it weren't for the fact that one day he met the woman who is now his wife, the woman he loves most in the world. They fell in love, had three children, and today they are happy together.

Although the happiness is never complete, although Collins adores his wife, takes care of her and even at the time he agreed with her and promised never to drink in this way again, today he is here, pouring rum again and with a pain in his heart. As he drinks the rum he feels guilt, he knows that he is disappointing his wife, that he is failing her. She would feel sad if she saw him drinking.

At the same time he feels anger, because his wife is the one who caused him to be there at this moment, Collins is hurt, he has been in a bad mood for days, he is grumpier than usual and those who know Collins know that the man is the noblest thing in the world, kind, respectful, always talking in a slow tone, without saying bad words and without attacking, but right now he is full of anger, now he cares very little about everything and that is why he asks for another drink from his favorite barman.

Think about how difficult it is for a man to be the head of the family, to always have a good attitude knowing that you have debts, that the mortgage is coming, that the child needs shoes, that the wife wants that dress, that two months ago you don't go to the park or the mall or to that attraction that came to town, these are so many things and as a father you want to fulfill them all like that, so don't even say thank you.

Collins has sought to comply and many nights he goes to bed proud of himself, of having complied like a good father, of having given his children what they needed and of smiling at feeling part of these achievements, that's what he thinks, that's what he feels.

What is the reason that brings Collins to this bar after fifteen years?

What happens every time he comes home, the being the good guy in the family, but the woman puts him in the place as the villain, and tells him that the boy did such a mischief, that she was waiting for him to scold him or that the other one broke the glass while playing with the ball.

Then, Collins, who came with the tiredness weighing on his soul, who was eager to get home, kiss his wife and stroke the children's hair to ask her how the day was going, has to put on his villain's face and scold the children for mischief that he doesn't even care about, He does it because that is what husbands have to do, to support each other, if he takes his wife's complaint as something frugal, then she will be angry for several

333

days, will tell him that she is alone for everything and the man will feel sad. He regrets so much that after a day of work he has to come to deal with things in the home that are his responsibility, he wonders what his wife's desire is to make him the villain, he is not the villain, he is the man who loves his children, the one who wants to play, once he came with the desire to play ball with the little one, to see how he was standing out, to take a few shots and to talk.

He was born as a father to do that and when his wife arrived, she told him that the little one had done a mischief and there was his prince, looking at him with a guilty face and Collins took out of where he did not have a rage to claim that mischief, he sent him to his room and was left with a heavy heart seeing his little one goes into his room, he had been left with the desire to play with him, with the desire to make him feel that he loved him, his wife did not even notice, she just wanted to get revenge and she got it.

That's why he drinks, because he doesn't want to go to that house where his wife waits for him with more complaints, claims, showing what he did or didn't do with a certain child, denying that such a child needs two straps, that the other one has to be punished, and he's there drinking because for days he has wanted to stay by the woman's side and yell at her to fuck off, that he's not a villain, that he doesn't have to make her beat the children for something she doesn't even care about. He wants to say it, but he is so angry that he prefers to control himself, he knows that if he opens his mouth he will scream, he will say bad words, he will hurt.

When he feels that the liquor is filling his head, he gets up, says goodbye to his lifelong bartender, and tells him that someday they will meet again. He leaves feeling the liquor in his head, today he didn't drink much, but so many years without stepping on this place besides the age he was, it was enough to make his mind foggy and get drunk faster than before.

A short time later he put the key in the door of his house, opened it, inside there was his wife, who was shouting something to one of the rooms, when she saw him, her greeting was:

—When he saw it, his greeting was: Thank goodness you've arrived, where were you? You have to scold that son of yours, he just gave me a bad face because I asked him to eat everything. Go and tell him something because he obeys you

—Why don't you make yourself obey then?

—How do you say?

—That I don't have to be the villain of the film that you can be.

—Do you think I don't spend all day putting them on the track, but they don't listen, they don't obey, only you.

—Make yourself respected.

—Do you smell liquor? —said his wife, making a sad face.

—Yes, I smell liquor, so what?

—You promised never to drink again.

—I'm fed up.

—Sick of what?

—Of coming to this house every day and having to put up with you making me mistreat the children, do you think I don't want to hug them? I want to play with them, not punish them, the problems they have had can be solved by you, you don't have to get me into that mess, if I come exhausted from work, with so many things on my mind, I don't have to add to that having to fight with my little ones, I just want to play.

—What are you talking about?

—I'm not going to scold my children anymore, not for things they haven't done to me.

That night Collins slept on the furniture, it was to be expected that his wife did not understand, although she lasted some days annoyed, at the worst she understood that she did not count on her husband to make them feel the authority and Collins did not return to the bar, every night he came home to play with his children and although the woman threw hints, he ignored them and enjoyed his little ones because he knew that in a sigh they would be gone, they would be with their own lives and he would have missed an important stage of their lives because of senseless fights invented by his wife.

Sometimes the parents are put as the villains to be able to raise the children and not always the parents want to be them, what more they wish in many occasions is to be able to arrive home to embrace their children and to rest for some hours of the hustle and bustle of the day.

Invasion

I am finally managing to gather the memories, what I had wanted so much for all this time, to have the complete stories to be able to publish them. Now as I write this, the voyeurist comes to mind who was watching the tenants of his hotel through a conduit, his whole hotel was for snooping, then Gay Talese would make a book about it and they made one of those stupid documentaries about the series.

I'm not a voyeurist who loves to watch sex, I had to do it because there was no other way out, but it's not because I like it, what I observe is human behavior, not what they do in a bed.

But I'm about to publish a book about what I've done these last years, nobody knows if it's the protagonist of the story, maybe you who read this if you feel identified, might think you were a victim of my field research work.

I'm going to tell you what I did and what I do. A few years ago I began to observe people in shopping malls, they all looked the same to me, like magazine clippings, they dressed alike, they laughed alike, the same types of families went and everyone acted the same way. They didn't have many differences and I noticed that as a pattern that would be interesting to investigate.

I searched for literature on the subject and didn't get much, except for psychological writings and Freud as a quote to support the nonsense they wrote. I spent a few months thinking about how I could properly investigate the case and the idea came to me without much planning, to invade their sites.

Of course, to enter their homes invading would break the habitat, but I did as those who observe the lions, who put themselves in the trees, camouflaged with mounts and spend days there, waiting for the perfect recording or photo. That's what I would do, I would get into these people's habitat without them noticing, and I would begin to review their behavior and document it.

How do I get into these places without being seen?

I dressed in black, settled down with some food, and went into the first house. I don't know why people in the suburbs are so trusting, leave a window open, or allow any corner to be snuck in. I got into the first house through a window, it was a short while before I knocked down a mountain of books with collections of nonsense all over them, but I didn't do it. I managed to get around it without a problem. I hid in a closet, behind some clothes, I was there for a few hours, how boring this is, being in this place makes me understand that I am still a novice in this, because while I am here, I realize that I did not bring a container to urinate in and I am squeezing, and then in the other visits I was more cautious and now, there may be an earthquake, to stay locked up and live until I am rescued.

In that first house, there was a married couple, a baby girl who was a bit spoiled, as it usually happens with only children. The man talked about work and named people I don't know who they were and when the girl left the room, I heard soft sounds, like the man caressing her and giving her kisses, something common in many of the houses I visited. That first time I had to stay locked up and listen to the couple's moans and the bed creaking, it was part of the documentary, I had to review it.

The next day they all came out, the first thing I did when I left that hiding place was to use their bathroom and pee with all the pleasure in the world.

Then, I planned to visit another house, this time with all the planning in the world. In this house, there was also a married couple, except that it was a boy they had and he was 9 years old, a boy who was almost a teenager. The man also pawed the woman and they talked nonsense, in this case, the leader of the pack was him. That day, in the hiding place where there was also a closet, I felt that the man entered the room, closed the door carefully and took out his cell phone, dialed and spoke to someone, a woman, said morbid words and that he loved her, then hung up quickly, that his wife was close by. He left as if nothing had happened. This pattern was so common in many homes that if I didn't like men so much I would seriously consider starting to date girls, infidelity is more common than we think.

In one house, a man lived alone, and I stayed there watching everything he did, seeing nonsense on his cell phone, seeing half-naked women and memes, that's where his life went.

My journey helped me to perfect the techniques of surveillance, because I did not want to just listen or intuit, I discovered that my body, small, could enter the air ducts, there I began to sneak, no one noticed and could watch in silence.

340

A pattern that I began to notice in many of the houses was the frugality with which people live, they are not planning anything to live tomorrow, I know they say you have to live now, but they only live it to do silly things, and they live tomorrow to worry about economic needs, deficiencies, and poverty.

Their economic limitations are focused on that, on thinking that they have, that they don't have, that they would like to. Women live with the illusion that they will be bought something, those who work show off their pride that they are workers, and I, who am a woman, can say that they look bad, because feminism comes to the surface, as if they were justifying themselves for what they do, men work and already, carefree with that, but women, show off their power, they have, they possess.

Imagine in those houses where they are the ones who work and the men stay at home. She imposes what has to be done, she is authoritarian, in one of those houses where I was, which are few, the woman told the man that that's why she worked and that she had to do what she said, that she was the authority and her rules were made, that's what her money was for. In short, machismo with a vagina. This type of woman made me think that many of us who defend feminism see our hands tied because this type of woman makes us look bad, shows us as figures who don't let anyone control us, and who loves to screw up.

I understand that for years we have been victims of many humiliations, of being second fiddle, even today that happens, but it doesn't give them any reason to behave that way, they make us look bad for what we are so hard to defend.

Among the fauna of people I met from the hiding place, I received curious images, such as the man who saw pictures of muscular men while his wife was sleeping next to him, or the boy hiding in his room wearing his sister's underwear. That same boy was talking about soccer with his father and seemed to be very masculine, I didn't want to be the disappointment for him, I also saw this subject a lot, people who had their intimate hiding places that didn't want the family to notice.

I also met men who had relationships with their maids and women who brought their lover when their husband left. I found many women who, when their husband left, would cry and some who, when they left, looked happier than when he was there. It was very common to encounter behavior from lonely people that they did not have when they were near their own, even children, who are honest, when they confirmed that they were alone, they did things that they would surely never do in the company, everyone responded mainly to curiosity.

In many homes, even in this century, I found women who were humiliated and beaten by men. I remember in one of the houses a man slapped the woman so hard that I jumped up and down, the man looked at where I was, his instinct told him something was there, but the woman was crying so hard that he concentrated on following her, for safety and for mental healing I went on my way to another place.

342

What I can say of all this is that my research made something clear, we are more alike than we think, even in different social strata, I was in the homes of people who barely had enough to eat, who were the most loving, I was in the homes of people who were millionaires who were living in hell and also the other way around.

I also confirmed that it doesn't matter the color of the skin, but everyone is either good or bad, but in many black communities I found solidarity, more loving and understanding men, the white one has a little more arrogance, I suppose because he feels superior for all these centuries, where he thinks he can go over the others that are not of his pigmentation or social stratum.

I also discovered that many people do not come out of the closet, that many others who look very serious have hidden things in the house that could surprise the most open-minded.

Many children are unhappy, although they do not even realize it themselves, and I also found that many people who live alone have less loneliness than many who live in the community, I found many houses with large families, where several in the home have a sadness that weighs heavily on them.

We human beings are similar and we still have a long way to go in order to change what we are. You can read all this in the book that will come out in two weeks where I tell my experience as a snooper in other people's homes.

The Neighbors

A few weeks ago, some neighbors moved in next to our house, the old house that had been abandoned for several years, and finally sold it. We saw the neighbors arrive, very nice, the man of the house approached me, he greeted me with that kindness of a newcomer and when he finished introducing himself he said that he was ready for whatever I needed. I found his offer strange, we are the ones who regularly offer this to newcomers, but I did not give it much importance.

The first few days nothing happened, we just listened to them dragging things around, making adjustments, some shouting from one of them so that the other would do something, some obscene word. That, there was nothing else in it. When the hustle and bustle ended, it was as if they had died, they were no longer heard, they did not speak, the footsteps and the screams were not heard, but one day, as if they had been resurrected, they began to speak, they woke me up in the morning, apparently talking while they were having breakfast, the dishes clashed, one shouted at the other what he wanted to drink, the other shouted to leave him and someone complained, a child cried and someone complained about it.

When they finished their breakfast they were silent, except for a few shouts, that was the theme, they talked to each other as if each one was on the top of a mountain and they had to shout to hear each other. That was tolerable, because being in the day to day, you can stand the noise, but at night they began to add noises that were frightening the sleep. I was afraid to

344

go to bed because I knew that as soon as I was getting sleepy they would start screaming like crazy people.

One night they added to their screams a dog, which began to bark, out of nowhere and did not shut up all night, barking, howling, and continuing to bark as if it had the lungs of a singer or trumpet player, there is nothing worse than a dog barking all night, out of nowhere, it shakes your sleep, adding to them laughter, screams, sounds of television that apparently no one was paying attention

This was going in a crescendo, the next night beside the dog, the screams, they started to put music, they put on rock metal, they changed to Latin songs, to Mexican songs that they chanted in a bad Spanish accent.

The weekends also turned into hell because added to the dog with big lungs, the screams, the music with a bass that made me jump on the bed, also the fights came, suddenly everything was silent, someone was screaming, a bottle was crashing against a wall, we were scared and then the screams and the blows of the flesh that was hurt with fists among those present.

So decent these people looked, incredible how they became and how bad neighbors they were.

I'm not one to make a fuss, I don't like it, my wife told me that we had to do something and pointed it out to me so that I would act, as I didn't want to get into trouble, she did act, got up, picked up the phone and dialed 911. She filed a report and soon after that, the police showed up. They talked, they pretended to be obedient and calm, she hadn't finished leaving when they made a noise again and I heard in one of the

345

shouts the man say bad words to the one who called 911.

The situation became more chaotic, they began to fight over various issues, but now they were not fighting alone in the house, outside, in the garden which was more like a pigsty where they had everything that could not fit inside, they had barbecues and we had to swallow all the smoke. When I came out and the man was wearing shorts, his hairy chest, and a lobster apron, he was yelling at me.

—Neighbor, how are you, a little meat?

—Thank you, I'm fine.

—Whenever you want, we are here to order, don't forget, you are welcome.

Again his offer, said with that seriousness, as if he was giving me a coded message, not super how to interpret this, I stayed thinking about his words, and again I reflected on what this person could be saying to me.

But the anger overcame what I could feel for this one and I went away insulting him in my mind, I wanted to end all of them, so many years of peace that we had had so that now the worst neighbors of the life arrived at us. I had never had such terrible neighbors as this one.

Sometimes we would all leave the house, as long as we didn't listen to their scandal, we would go to the mall, to the bustle of this place, people walking around, music, bargains, and other noises. We would arrive close to the night with the hope of finding peace, but already from a distance, I could see that all their lights were on, that you could see the shadows going from one side to the other, crossing with their screams. One woman was shouting to her husband to go upstairs, that something had happened to the kitchen tap, another one was saying that the water in the shower was freezing, that he should repair it. The man, who always greeted me so receptively, hurled an insult-laden with bad vibes.

You would think that this couldn't be worse, but yes, and I discovered it, the model family that lived next door to us gave it some reforms, some reforms that seemed long, because one morning my head woke up jumping in blows, in the house next door they were hammering, while they listened to music at full volume, it was blows, shouts, other blows, change of songs. It is worth saying that it was barely six-fifty in the morning. I drank my coffee with a stitch in my head that promised to turn into a migraine.

How to solve this, our house could not be abandoned, we were still paying the mortgage. Calling the police was useless, they kept making noise, they didn't pay attention, they were such terrible neighbors that once my wife called to file a report and they said it was useless, that they paid the fines that they didn't give a damn if they were reported, that we could take the problem to court. I considered it, but that man scared me, I don't know why, but I was afraid of him, I guess my other neighbors felt the same way and that's why we hadn't ended up in court.

Several days with the same thing, beatings, insults, complaints, falling debris, my house vibrating, not to mention the dust that began to come in, sneaking in through the windows and objects, the renovation was intense, but it was worse when they started working with wood and chopping and sanding it on-site, everyone in the house was allergic and there wasn't a single object that didn't have a brown dust film on it.

My wife would grumble and insult them, telling me that I was a coward for not going to solve this, that those neighbors would end our marriage, because she didn't plan to live her whole life like that, that she would go to her mother's in Chicago, on the other side of the country. I believed her, she looked more upset than ever, she had to get the solution out of them. I was tired of these neighbors who didn't let me sleep, who had us all in a bad mood. This was a collective problem, but for some reason, the acoustics were directed at us and although the other neighbors heard them it was less intense than how we heard them, that is, I heard it softer. We did feel the screams as if they were next to us, we were in the same house.

Other neighbors didn't even know about the renovation, some were suspicious because they saw the materials arrive, not because of anything else. But they were fine with that neighbor, one more, who just made a little noise, but it was all a matter of getting used to it, that's why they didn't call 911.

One day, I go out and find my dear neighbor going through some of his yard waste, it seemed that he was looking for something among the missing objects he had in that driveway. What looked most like his house was the house of the drug addicts who collect garbage in the garden.

I don't know if these neighbors were drug addicts, but from their behavior, I wouldn't be surprised. When the neighbor sees me, he stops what he was doing and looks at me, raises his hand with a wide smile, and greets me, and wishes me a good day. His smile looks sincere, needy as if he is telling me that I have to go, that he is waiting for me there.

That day I drove away and thought about the words of that neighbor. What was his eagerness to have me visit him? Something that also made me curious was that although I was sure he had many people living at home, I could only remember his wife that I saw her passing by and he was clear about it, but the children, the family that lived in that house I had never seen, I had heard, many voices seemed familiar, but I could not relate to a face.

One night, when they were louder than ever and my wife was walking around, I decided to do what I should have done a long time ago, knock on her door and tell her to stop screwing around once and for all, to come down and yell at her, that it was three in the morning and that if she wanted to avoid an affair with me she should shut her mouth once and for all.

I went resolutely to his garden, opened the gate, walked to the entrance and knocked, the front door opened and there was no one inside. I passed by, and the house had a lot of belongings, but I didn't see a single person. I shouted to the man, I went upstairs, I went to the rooms and in that house, there was no noise or life, I was getting scared, but when I got to the bathroom that had a huge mirror and I saw my face, that was the new neighbor, I understood everything, I was my neighbor.

The Cat

He lived alone, since he had left his parents' house he sought to be alone in a house where he set his own rules and adapted to his own conditions, the truth is that Trevor was not a man to be in a good mood, regularly when he was spoken to he responded in a derogatory manner, it is not that he was a bad person, he did not wish him harm, he simply did not like to share with anyone, he did not pick on others and did not want them to pick on him.

The man was very quiet, his house was full of books on each of the walls, wherever he walked you would find a tower with texts of all kinds, from famous stories to silly literature, he would read whatever fell into his hands. His house didn't have a TV, there were no streaming subscriptions of any kind, except for the guilty pleasure of a YouTube channel that had classical music and exclusive content for fans, he followed it so he could enjoy new compositions, remastering, and information about concerts in the city. His law of being alone all the time didn't want it to be broken by anyone when in some event he flirted with a woman, he took her to a hotel, where they had their meetings and then followed their paths, and this he did more out of social commitment and physiological need than the pleasure that an ordinary man has in being with some woman.

One day, coming home from the bookstore with the new acquisitions that had arrived in the country, he found a black cat sitting in the middle of the door, staring at it and looking like it was waiting for him, Trevor looked at it for a few seconds and the cat grunted. Gently moving it with his foot, the cat stood up and took a few steps to the side, with its tail raised. Trevor went inside and ignored the animal, thinking that maybe it was from the street and was there looking for food or looking for a life.

The next day, when he went out to the fruit shop, he found the cat at the door, when he saw it, he grabbed it again, this time he didn't push it and passed it on the side. He went to get the groceries and when he came back he was there. He opened the door and the cat, without being invited, entered his house. This was a crime for Trevor, who passed by and began to tell him in a violent tone that he had to leave immediately, he thought of a dirty animal, urinating his books, chewing the leaves, messing up his papers, filling everything with hair, the animal was smart, because he climbed up to the highest column of books and there he stayed by looking at it and yanking when he saw it.

Trevor looked for the broom and wanted to shake it, without hurting it, it was not to attack animals, the animal dodged it and got off, ran after it, grabbed it, and threw it out into the street.

He went to bed quietly, opened the duty book, and read until he was drunk with sleep. He slept peacefully, as he did every night. He woke up because he felt a noise in the room, as he looked for the origin it was the cat that was taking a bath with its tongue when the looks met the animal grunted. He approached him to get the animal out and this time the animal did not even try to run away. He took it, took it out of the house and looked for the place where it entered, he didn't find the place until the afternoon, when he thought he could

352

pass through the roof, through the hole in the attic. He couldn't find any other way.

That day when he went out to do some shopping he didn't see the cat anywhere, he breathed a sigh of relief that he didn't have to keep dealing with a problem so silly that it seemed to start getting complicated. When he returned, he understood why the animal was not outside, sleeping on top of one of his book towers. He looked at it for a while and thought that the cat was not bad at all, it was black, like Poe's, he seemed to have chosen it as his slave, because it would not leave him alone, nor because he had taken it out of the house several times. He didn't say anything to the animal and went to the corner, where there was a pet store, bought a bag of food of the brand recommended and a bag of sand with a container, came home, installed it and the animal behaved as if it had been there all its life, started using the sandbox and eating, a couple of days later Trevor was reading a book and the cat was sleeping on the side, quiet, a couple of lonely companions who shared the roof and life.

Everything would seem to be going smoothly, if he hadn't noticed something strange about the animal, there were days when it would disappear, you couldn't see it anywhere and the food would get soft and the water slimy, it would simply vanish, he read on the internet that this was normal, that cats used to sneak around for several days, especially when they felt that there was a cat in heat nearby, that would surely come back as Rocky, bruised and limping, but happy to have sown the seed in some cat.

That did not happen, in fact, the animal returned, but it arrived as if nothing had happened, beautiful and gallant as always, he did not see it arrive, he simply appeared one morning in the house, he was grooming himself and meowed as soon as he saw it. Trevor caressed him for a while behind his ears and the animal began to purr, they greeted each other after an absence of several days.

For several days the cat was at home, eating, doing its own thing, and then getting close to it. Trevor would read some books and every now and then he would give the animal a treat. The cat was no longer on the floor, but climbed onto the bed and now that double mattress was shared by him and the cat.

Trevor got used to the presence of the cat, he even needed it, he discovered it one morning when he woke up and the animal was not there, what he missed most was that even though he looked for the place where the cat was escaping, he did not find it, the animal went in and out somewhere he did not know. His house was closed, he had a couple of windows in the living room, with sliding windows that were always closed and with the lock on, the door was solid wood, without pet doors, in the kitchen he had an equally solid door, the second one had some windows and all of them were closed.

It was winter and he kept everything closed, he looked in the basement and he couldn't find a way out either and went to the attic and realized that it was impossible for the animal to enter or leave there, simply because the cat, no matter how agile it was, couldn't jump into that small place, at most a rat would fit in and that cat was big.

354

Trevor could not concentrate on reading, some-times he would reach out to pet the animal, but it was not there and left his reading because he wondered where the little animal was and worse when it would return. What he did not want happening. He started sleeping badly thinking about the cat and also getting in a bad mood, he lived alone precisely to avoid attachments and suffering for others, every living being was an independent soul that had to be in his space, he could not mess with another one because it would destabilize it.

Almost a month passed and the cat did not appear, Trevor started to investigate, went out and started to check in neighboring houses from outside, to see if his cat was one of those scoundrels that had two houses, who ate a little in one and another and thus gave themselves a better life than kings, but he did not find that any neighbor had a black cat. She returned home hoping to find him there, but he wasn't there either. The animal was nowhere to be seen, it was as if it had disappeared.

Two months after the cat left, it appeared, as always, hungry, and beautiful, Trevor noticed the cat because it jumped on the bed and started meowing for food and affection, he with all the joy went and served its food, he was happy that the animal had returned, he was with it all the time and at night he closed the room with the cat, knowing that inside it was literally impossible for the cat to escape, he would not allow it to leave again. For several months the relationship was normal, between master and cat, it ran around the house, they shared and it was the most loved cat of all.

But then the animal disappeared again, and it did so in the middle of the night, with the room closed. When Trevor woke up and did not find the animal, he turned his room upside down, checked every corner, but there was nothing, it was impossible for it to have escaped in spite of the fact that it opened the door and went out again.

It was missing for several months, during which time Trevor was in sadness, waiting for the animal every day, and when it finally appeared, he attended to it with great joy. If anyone had seen from a window, they would have found a gray man, in his house, thin and holding a book with his fingers halfway up and caressing the air, next to a jar of food that no animal used.

The Baby

Tiffany didn't like children, she had it clear since she was a child, when she had to endure helping to raise her younger brothers and also cousins, she said that in her adolescence she had exhausted her patience to raise children, so when she reached her sexual age she protected herself with a lot of dedication not to get pregnant. She didn't want an accident to happen and have to ruin her body by creating life.

With her boyfriends, several of them had no problem with the issue of having children. They were happy not to have to deal with the romance of a woman they loved and got pregnant. But finally, there was this man who fell in love with her, who made her float and made her feel loved. Everything was going smoothly, but one day they fell into the children's conversation, he brought him out, who said that when they had a baby they were going to name him Matthias, because that's what his grandfather called himself, Tiffany looked at him up and down, surprised by the man's determination and told him to forget, that she would never have children. The boyfriend thought it was something she was saying to get out of the way, to fill the space, but then he realized that her foundation was solid and that she was determined not to have children, that she was not even determined to adopt him, she was simply determined not to get pregnant.

When she was 25 years old, she started to work on not having children definitively, she went to her gynecologist and told him that she wanted to have her fallopian tubes removed, to have them tied so that she

357

would never have a child. The doctor told her that she was insane, that he couldn't do that to her, that she was an active woman and could change her mind, that it wasn't allowed, but Tiffany was so insistent that the doctor chose to give her the card of a psychiatrist friend of hers so that they could talk about the "problem" that day. The doctor lost a high-value client because she decided never to set foot in that caveman's office again.

She went to other doctors, but the answer was almost the same, she tried doctors, to see if women understood each other better, but her luck didn't change, the gynecologists looked like mother hens and the medicine didn't allow her to hook up until she had at least three children or a risk to her health, so what Tiffany decided to do was to keep looking for a doctor and talk more openly about a bribe. Several of them took her out of the office and called her crazy, but she tried so hard that she finally found a doctor who would perform the procedure. This was a doctor who was gay by all accounts, but a loving, loving and understanding person, who identified with her and told her that between the two of them they left the secret that she had a disease in one of her tubes, that it was time to intervene immediately to prevent cancer. This was done, and a couple of months later Tiffany was safely on her way to pregnancy.

When she found another boyfriend, she talked to him about what she had done, from the beginning, to get her off the cloud if she thought she would get pregnant and have children like the typical American movie.

She began to live her life, already relieved to know that in this life she would not get pregnant, knowing that she would not have to raise more children. But luck spat in her face when one day one of her cousins showed up at her door, the woman looked exhausted, as if she had weeks without sleep. She came to bring him the bad news that his sister had died a month earlier. Tiffany was not the most homely, so they had this estrangement, although she was surprised they didn't tell her about her little sister's death, she had suffered from cancer that had eaten her up in a few weeks. She didn't have time for anything. This would be a hard blow for her, she loved her sister and would always regret not being able to say goodbye.

But the worst thing was not that, along with her sister's death there was a letter:

Little sister, life takes me, I will not be able to finish raising my little Jacob, I know that you, will raise him with all the love that my prince deserves. I love you, thank you for being my sister and guide.

Along with the letter came a six-month-old baby who was crying at the time with a high-pitched scream and wouldn't even look at her.

They both felt the rejection of each other and so she did not take him in her arms even though it was the right thing to do. She took the baby as if she had just picked up a bag of something that disgusted her or was a great danger, carried the little one to a bed and left it there, the baby continued crying and her first one vanished, as if relieved to be rid of that child.

The little one cried for a long time and in the end, apparently tired, he fell asleep. Tiffany sat up in front of the bed and looked at that child and wondered what she had gotten herself into, what crime she had committed so that the universe would mock her in the face and bring her that baby.

In the little one's bag came a series of instructions, she thought of her sister and began to read them, the hours when she should give her food, how to prepare the baby food and the type of crying along with the need, how much she had to change the diaper, when she was hungry, in pain or wanted love. According to her sister, the crying now was apparently a desire to have her bottom wiped. The baby was dirty, a great way to debut as a mother.

She put on a mask and started doing her homework, cleaning it up. She opened the diaper and found that little surprise, a yellow mass with a strong smell.

—How could such a small child do that? —He said before he choked on the vomit, he gagged several times, but he managed to hold on. He cleaned the baby, but felt he hadn't done enough. He didn't like children, but he wasn't a monster not to clean up well.

It was because of the note sheet, where she gave details of how to bathe him and she realized that it was a big job to wash a baby's ass, she followed the steps as recommended by her sister and bathed him, although with a lot of anxiety because while she was holding him in the bathroom, she felt that the little one was getting out of hand, In fact, a couple of times she slipped and went to the bottom of the water, took it out and cried disconsolate and terrified because she had swallowed water, when she finished, she dried it, dressed it and left it there, clean, she lay down next to it, exhausted, she felt that she had run fifty kilometers, she saw the baby making little sounds and looking at her, she moved her little arms and feet and she began to fall asleep.

The crying woke her up, she stood up again and went for the instructions, it was hunger, how the hell she prepared a teapot. Her sister's instructions were ambiguous, she prepared the water, the milk and put it in the teapot, she didn't screw it up properly and as soon as she tipped the container over the baby, the suck and the lid came off, everything fell over the little one who, terrified, started crying again. It was time to start over, bathe him, clean him up, Tiffany sat down to cry, frustrated because she had no idea what to do. When she calmed down, she got up, undressed the little boy, cleaned him with wet towels and dressed him again, prepared the teapot again and this time she made sure to close it well, put it in the little boy's mouth and he started to suck, but immediately he cried, he did not understand what was wrong with him, why this little boy did not stop crying, he checked it, smelled it and then realized that the teapot was on fire, he had burned it, he had to wait a little bit to be able to give it to him, but he rejected it again, after investigating for a while he knew that he had not sweetened it.

Finally, she fed the little boy and fell asleep. She also fell asleep, with her mouth open, exhausted. She didn't know what time it was, but she woke up, the baby was crying loudly, was hungry or in pain. She offered him food and he refused it, checked his diaper, realized he had put it on backward, put it back, but the baby was crying. She read the instructions from top to bottom and realized that the only thing that could be happening was that she hadn't gotten the gas out of the little one, she touched him on his tummy and felt it hard, she started to massage him, following her intuition and some gas came out, the little one calmed down and went back to sleep, she too, some time later she cried again, this time from hunger.

The next day Tiffany was just a woman's rag, she took care of the baby in a less disastrous way but she realized that her life had changed, she seriously considered taking the baby to home and leaving him in a basket just like he was in the movies, that some fat nuns were in charge of raising that child, that she had not tied her tubes in vain, but she could not break her sister's last will, she could not fail herself in that way, she was her little sister, her dear sister who was hurting her, by the way, the little one was the same face like her, so it hurt even more.

What she thought then was to take care of her for a while. She talked to the family to have them take care of the baby, all her family knew that she was not a lover of babies, she began to obey her sister's guidelines and call all the relatives to tell them to take care of the baby, but not one offered to help her with the little one, they all had strong excuses.

Months passed and Tiffany found herself some nights watching the baby's sleep and realizing how he was growing, keeping details to himself, buying him toys, and starting to have the habits of a mother. As cold as she was with the babies, they bonded, became attached to each other, and smiled willingly and bitterly on the day the little one said, mommy.

362

Sometimes the ironies of life are dirty, mauve, and unhappy.

The Cloud

As a child he loved to lie down in the meadow and watch the sky, he could spend the whole afternoon looking at the clouds and finding shapes, he would see the one that looked like a chicken, the one that looked like a painting, the one that looked like a turtle or a dinosaur, the one that looked like something scatological or the one that looked like a relative.

His afternoon would pass until his mother called him to come in for dinner. He was always a lonely child and enjoyed these moments to explore and to blow his mind. That's why he would build stories with the clouds, who would look at him, who would have conversations with them. He still remembers when he saw the first version of The Lion King, when he saw Simba's father talking from the cloud, he knew that those white things in the sky were more than smoke collecting rain, that they meant a spiritual connection with human beings.

Thomas grew up and got married, had a couple of children, and worked in a company where he could stay for many years until he retired, had the typical American life, normal, without many ups and downs.

When his first son was old enough to understand, he showed him the first cloud, they laid down in the garden and he started showing him the clouds, he associated them with everything he had seen in his short life, the stuffed animal he liked, the little turtle in the YouTube song or his mother, sometimes he had such a big imagination that he could guess at the shapes of the clouds, objects that were more developed than he could believe.

Soon it would be a family game, they would see the clouds from time to time, and the game was all about finding the craziest shape and having reasons, it wasn't worth inventing.

The years passed and the children grew up, and life became calmer at home when they left, they still had a few years left to retire. He worked because he kept himself alive.

One day, driving along the highway, she saw a cloud on top, it was almost dusk, then the sun's rays hit her and gave her a pinkish hue, she was shaped like a cartoon elephant, you could even see the hole in her little eye and a long thread that was the trunk.

He smiled and wanted one of his children to be there so he could show him the cloud, he wanted to take a picture of it, but he was going on the highway, it was not wise to take out his cell phone, it could crash. The next day, when he left on his way to work he found the cloud, only now it was not pink, but white, he thought it was strange to see it there, positioned in the same place, the only thing he could think about it was that it was a little fog, but maybe he did not find a sense that this cloud was there, there was nothing in science that explained this event.

When he went out in the afternoon, he drove away and hung in the sky, there he found the cloud, it was pink again, and it seemed to be watching him. He was so impressed that he had to put his foot on the brake until the end because he was a few millimeters away from hitting a Lexus, which was behind him, almost hitting him.

He had to control himself, was breathing, calm, trying to calm the anxiety that was a product of the scare that had just happened and that cloud that was watching him, driving looking at the cloud and at the same time pending the road. When he got home he had no contact with the place where the cloud was, so he couldn't know if it was there or not.

The next day he saw it again and advanced to an open space where people were going to change tires or repair the car, he got out and began to observe the cloud, in detail, he took out his mobile and zoomed in to see it better, it looked normal, like any cloud, even in case he compared it with another one, he zoomed in and took pictures of both, to be able to see them from the computer in the office, he was willing to reveal what was going on with that cloud, why he was still there, why he was watching his every move and was alert to what he was doing, well, that's what he was starting to think, that that cloud was there for him, watching his movements, was something of the third type, or that he could only see himself.

That day when he returned, his wife accompanied him, he had his car repaired and would be ready until Friday, then on his way back he showed her the cloud that also had the pink tones.

—Do you see that cloud?

—Which one? It's pretty, it looks like a pink elephant.

366

—Would you believe me if I told you that it has been there for several days?

—That's impossible, a cloud always seems to be moving. It can't stay static.

—I've been seeing it for days, and it looks at me, it has something against me.

His wife looked at him strangely, as if she were beside a madman.

—What are you talking about, love? It's a cloud, and maybe you thought so, or the shape of that mountain where you see it, generates some effect that makes the cloud have that shape, I don't know, it has to have an explanation, it's not going to be something strange, don't tell me that now after you're old you'll get those crazy ideas.

The man didn't stay with that one, he didn't want to investigate just because, he seemed crazy, the next day he went and saw the cloud, he tried not to see it, he put the radio on and listened to varied songs until work, controlling his anxiety so as not to lose control of the car.

During the rest of the week, he saw the cloud, so on the weekend he went to the mountain, prepared everything, drove as far as the road allowed and got out, there, on the side of the mountain you could see the cloud, immense, that was watching him, who seemed happy because he had finally heard the call and was on his way to see it.

The road was steep, difficult, but little by little he climbed up and the cloud seemed to have more shape. As he approached the beginning of the cloud the sun's rays began to paint it pink. He reached a part of the road, where in order to cross he would have to take a huge jump of more than 200 meters, he walked, bordered that small abyss and saw in the distance a wooden bridge that reminded him of the bridge from one of the Indiana Jones movies, the one that is released and almost throws Indi into the void. He started to cross it, a wind current swayed the bridge that creaked like rotten wood, he was now closer to the cloud and as he crossed it holding on tightly, he saw that the cloud had turned inside it, as if it was alive, as if he was happy to see it and wanted it soon by his side.

He finally reached the other side, just at the moment when a strong current of air caused the bridge to end and took the bridge away. A small wave of panic ran through the man, who felt cold and thought about how he would return, but he looked at the cloud and knew that nothing else mattered, going down to earth would be easy, the hardest work had been accomplished, being close to the cloud.

He walked towards it, it was so big that you couldn't see the end, just a pink mist that was wrapping the whole environment, like when an airplane goes through clouds in the air. Soon it was difficult to see where he was stepping, the atmosphere was so pink and so dense that he could not see anything, each step was given carefully, not to go to find a cliff and die there, lost in that mountain.

As he went in, he felt an incredible peace, he knew that this cloud had called him, that he had to be there, and the stress of the previous days was gone, the fears, the worries, the anger, everything, was in an immense peace that for a moment he wondered if he was dying and this was the peace that those who came back to life after seeing the so-called white light talked about so much.

But no, he was alive and the cloud asked him to walk, he did so, he followed his core, the vortex that swirled around like a whirlpool in the center and that was the final destination for him, for a moment he felt that his feet did not step on anything. He felt a terrible sensation in his stomach, like when elevators move strongly, but he did not fall, he was inside the cloud, he walked, confident in that pink elephant, he finally arrived at the nucleus, the peace was total, he closed his eyes and the wind caressed his face, his senses seemed absent until now, he had not realized that in all this time his senses were not the same, they seemed attenuated.

With his eyes closed he began to feel every sensation in his body, the body, the smells, the sounds, everything seemed to return. He felt an immense peace, but he no longer felt in the midst of the clouds, he was in another place, he did not want to open his eyes, the sounds seemed strange and at the same time familiar. He breathed several times, softly, as when he was meditating, he opened his eyes and a white light made him close them again, he heard voices of alarm, of joy, of surprise. When her eyesight adjusted, she saw herself on top of a hospital bed, her whole family was by her side, excited.

The doctors came in to check him, took his pulse, put lights in his eyes, and did tests. Hours later, when his mind had adjusted, he knew he had been in a coma for a year. They didn't turn him off because he had hoped; he had had an accident after he saw a beautiful elephant-shaped cloud on his way home.

The Promotion

Lori has been waiting for a promotion for more than six years, and it hasn't quite arrived yet. She has been an unimpeachable worker, the bosses have told her, in every company where she has been. In the office where she has worked for more than ten years, she has not been promoted, but she has had a change of bosses, she goes from the Finance office to Accounting, to Marketing and always the assistant to all the managers of the company and each one of them knows that she is the best thing that could have happened in the company because she knows the vibration of each area, how it is done, the clients, the suppliers and what has to be done. They all recognize that she alone could take care of the company if she had enough hands to do the immensity of the work.

Although everyone knew it, they did not give her the promotion that she wanted so much, to be executive manager, below the general manager, a position where she would earn a very substantial salary and at the same time have another series of benefits, such as company car, insurance, longer vacations, benefits for her children and everything that is expected in large companies that take care of their employees.

She felt somewhat frustrated, some nights she could not sleep well, because her desire to be a manager was seen only as a dream, she had done everything in her power to achieve it, now the only thing left was to let go, let Providence decide whether she deserved that promotion or not.

Sometimes, when attachments to things are generated, one suffers when they do not materialize, resentments and anger appear because they do not give you what you think you deserve. That happened to Lori, she respected her bosses a lot, she was fond of them, that affection that is generated in the work offices, where co-workers and bosses are respected and loved. But at the same time, every time she saw the manager of a certain area, she felt anger, it caused her to shout that she deserved the promotion, that why did they wait so long to give it to her, that if she had to sleep with someone to get it, that if she was twenty years younger, with a more upright ass and the prettiest tits, they would give it to her, all that she thought while she smiled sweetly at her boss and asked him if he needed anything else.

But the same Providence to which Lori was releasing everything, knew that the moments are written and everything comes when it has to come, finally she was given the miracle, one Friday she was called to the meeting room, as soon as she entered she found all her bosses, each of the managers. At the top was the owner, the boss of bosses, an old man who looked at her with tenderness and sweetness, she said:

—In all my business life I have never had the honor of having an employee like you, who learned to blend in with every area, who knew how to face challenges no matter how big, you could do the job better than this old man.

—How can you think of it, you are an eminence.

372

—You remind me of myself when I was young. I admire you so much. Can you imagine why we brought you here?

She smiled and said.

—I think so.

Everyone laughed at Lori's innocent response.

—Yes, it's what you imagine, from this Monday you'll be working under me, managing all the points, your life is going to change completely from now on. Are you ready?

—"For a long time," said Lori with a joy that couldn't fit on her chest.

The other managers started applauding and congratulating her. The meeting closed with a toast. They recommended that she go shopping for the weekend, she had, without knowing it, a special bonus in her bank account to go buy dresses and suits because now she would have to go out a lot, meet with businessmen, with people in the middle, go to cocktail parties and she had to show the image of the company, the position had many benefits, but also a large number of responsibilities.

That weekend along with her husband they went to several shopping malls and lived for a day the dream of every woman, go to many stores, buy the most expensive and knowing that she would use it several times and would look splendid, the husband all day must have been sitting, supporting or giving thumb down when he did not like a suit, the back of the car was full of bags from many luxury stores, it was a life of rich people who had given themselves that day.

On Sunday they went for a walk in the country, ate, and spent the rest with the family, which was the introduction to Lori's new life. She was immensely happy, proud of achieving that position for which she had worked so hard. The story of her promotion was the talk of the town and the family called to congratulate her.

On Monday she arrived, she put on the dress she liked best, and when she thought she should go out, her cell phone rang, it was a man with an educated voice who spoke to her as Doña Lori and told her that outside he was waiting for her. As she left, a black Lexus, a luxury car, which she had only seen when her boss, the owner, had arrived, was now looking for her.

She went out, the driver, dressed in a custom-made suit opened the door and greeted her with much cordiality. She got into the car and was surrounded by many luxuries, when she arrived at the office all her colleagues received her with congratulations and joy, they knew nothing, they barely knew.

So much for Lori's celebration, who now began to pay for the high position she had, that night, after the office work where she was catching up with her responsibilities, she had to go to a company event, she left with what she considered her best gala. When she left, she was approached by the press, who quickly interviewed her and asked her why she thought she had been elected to that position, whether she felt capable of achieving it because of her status as a woman since no woman had ever held that important position before. That would be her first mistake because the journalist brought out her yellow side and the next day the headline was New Manager does not tolerate comments contrary to her way of thinking, it seems that her condition as a woman will limit good decisions, is the company safe?

The other mistake was in the meeting, which did not know how to behave with the label and also some men did not take it as seriously as they deserved for the same reason, being a woman.

For several days she had to start earning her place in the workplace, to give herself credit, to be respected for what she was, for that value she had and that she had trained in the company for years, but in this environment in which she was, it was difficult for her to prove that as a woman she had everything to gain, to show that she could be even better than the men.

Little by little, Lori learned to position herself as a leader in her environment, to step up and give herself respect. There is no denying that in the beginning, when she started working in her new position, she had to suffer through the nights without sleep because the next day she would have important meetings, like the one she would have with a Chinese man, or Russians, Indians and other businessmen from outside who had ingrained machismo, and seeing a woman in such a high position was almost an insult.

She managed to settle in, little by little, like what she wanted, when the businessmen trampled on her, her answers were so categorical that this businessman looked at her with skepticism, smiled, agreed with her, and went on.

Over the years, her position was recognized in the media, everyone knew that she was a strong businesswoman who deserved respect, and the more macho ones said that she was a man who was born in a woman's body, and the less macho ones said that she was a woman with a more solid temperament than any man and that they would negotiate with her with their eyes closed.

As for the home, the change of position affected it a bit, because from going back and forth during office hours, the woman went from never being at home to having countless events in the day and sharing with people of all kinds and all nationalities.

But she knew how to get around, her family learned to adapt to the change and now they live in another social stratum, happy, integrated, and adapted as they always wanted.

Being an entrepreneur in a time when even men dominate the world can be difficult to digest for many.